A HOT LINE TO YOUR HORSE

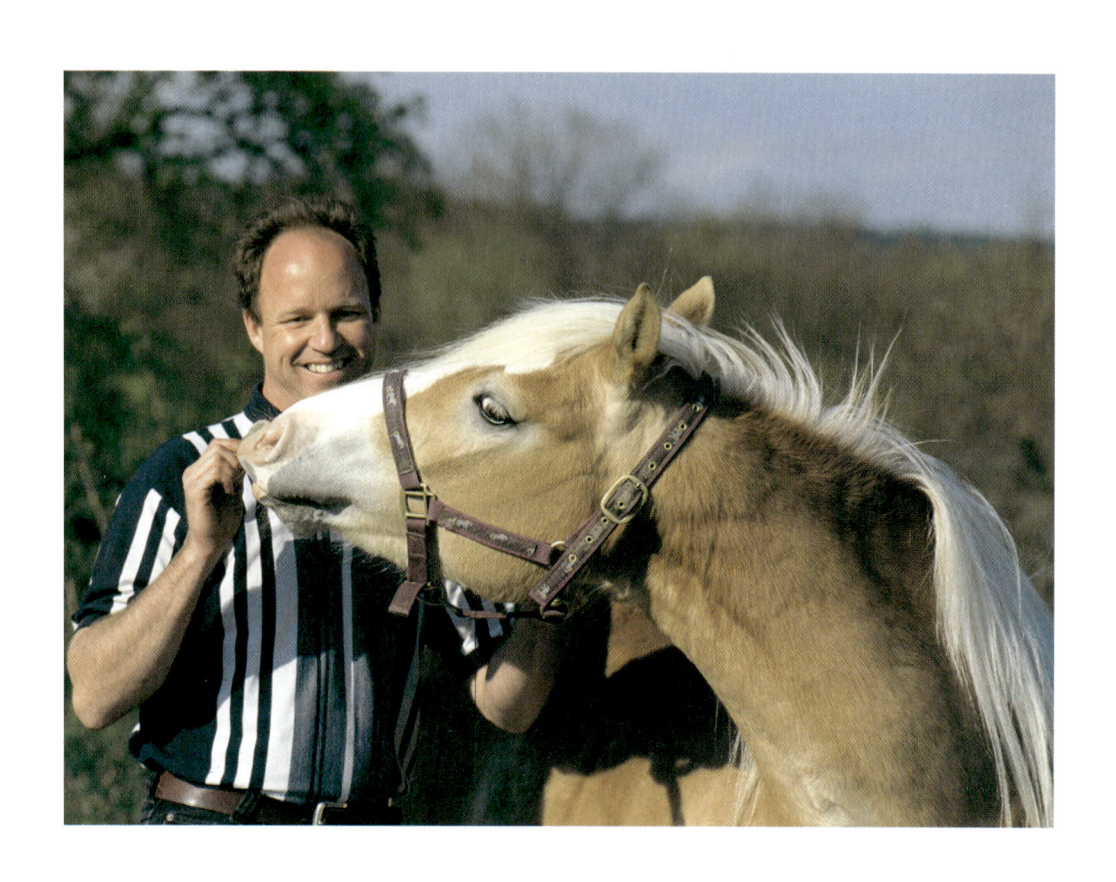

A HOT LINE TO YOUR HORSE

A PRESSURE POINT SYSTEM
FOR SOLVING MUSCLE PROBLEMS

Chris Olson

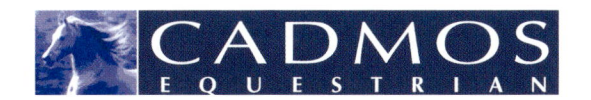

CADMOS
EQUESTRIAN

Copyright of original German edition © 1997/2000 by Cadmos, Lüneburg
Copyright of this edition © 2002 Cadmos Equestrian
Photos: Christiane Slawik
Translated by Desiree Gerber
Typesetting and design: Ravenstein + Partner
Printer: Westermann, Zwickau
All rights reserved.
Reproduction or storage of this publication by or in any
electronic medium is forbidden without the written
permission of the publisher.
Printed in Germany
ISBN 3-86127-901-0

CONTENTS

1. ABOUT MY WORK ... 6

2. AROUND THE PRESSURE POINT SYSTEM 11
2.1. Muscles – where tension starts.... ..12
2.2. Eliminating tension in muscles.... ..16
2.3. Fingertips and more 17
2.4. Safety precautions 19
2.5. Feel the difference!............ ..20

3. JUST ONE SINGLE TENSED-UP MUSCLE BUT ... 24
3.1. The elastic band 25
3.2. The spinal column 26
3.3. Joint damage................. ..29

4. PHYSICAL RELAXATION: THE PRESSURE POINT SYSTEM (PPS) 30
4.1. The first test................. ..34
4.2. The eight regions of the pressure point system 35
   4.2.1. Region 1 35
   4.2.2. Region 2 39
   4.2.3. Region 3 42
   4.2.4. Region 4 45
   4.2.5. Region 5 50
   4.2.6. Region 6 53
   4.2.7. Region 7 54
   4.2.8. Region 8 55
4.3. The concluding test............ ..59
4.4. When and how often should you use PPS?........... ..58
4.5. Extended reference to the individual regions........ ..58
   4.5.1. Region 1 59
   4.5.2. Region 2 59
   4.5.3. Region 3 60
   4.5.4. Region 4 61
   4.5.5. Region 5 62
   4.5.6. Region 6 62
   4.5.7. Region 7 63
   4.5.8. Region 8 63

5. ADDITIONAL INFORMATION AND GYMNASTIC EXERCISES FOR YOUR HORSE 65
5.1. The warm-up in connection with PPS..................... ..67
5.2. Important and often forgotten: cooling down 68
5.3. Exercises to build the muscles 69
5.4. Stretching: useful gymnastic exercises for your horse 72
5.5. The carrot trick................ ..75

CONCLUSION 79

1. ABOUT MY WORK

The author

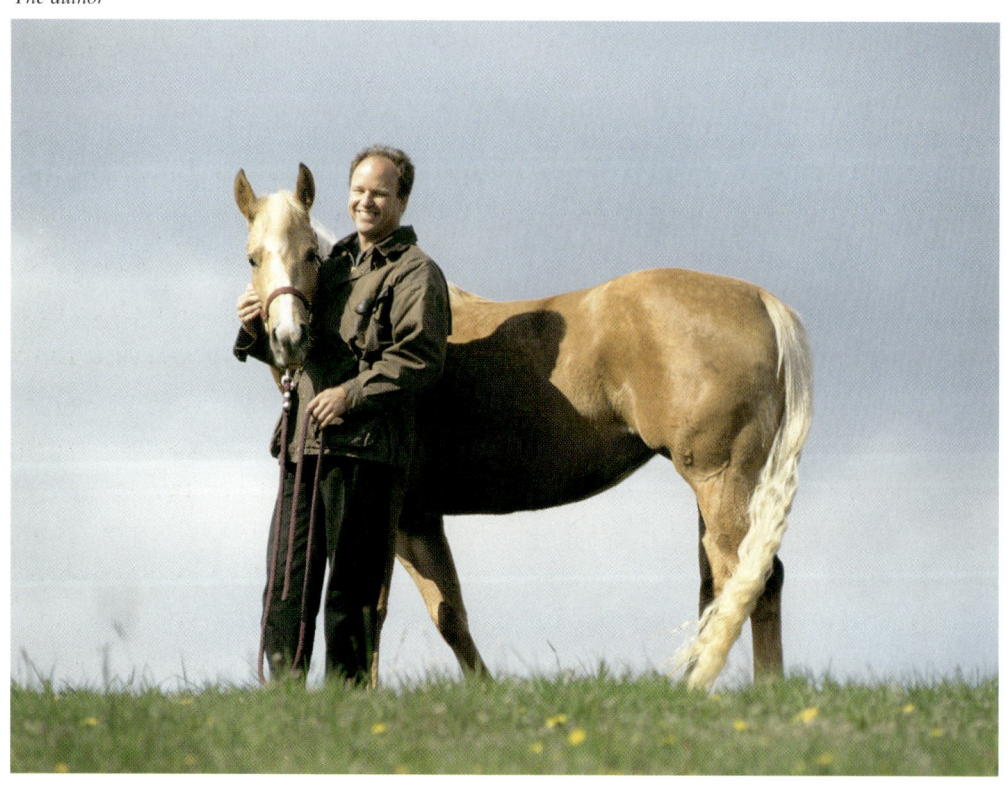

About my work

Tension in horses often causes loss of performance and impairs harmonious cooperation between horse and rider. You almost certainly know of such problems and would like to avoid them. This book is intended to help. Maybe you will find some of the methods a bit unusual, but I promise you they are successful, without you or your horse having to take any risks.

I have worked with horses for a long time. I am now trying, by using the pressure point system to deal with extensive areas of physical and emotional stress, to develop an effective, easily comprehensible method to enhance the well-being and willingness to perform of our four-legged friends. This method of massage stimulates the nervous system and promotes well-being in your horse.

I have tried in particular to find an easily understood system, capable of being simply described in clear terms.

Using my method, every horse owner can master the extensive and often confusing pressure point system, so that at the very least the well-being of your horse will be improved. I will help you every step along the way.

Being a flight animal the horse has to rely on a well-functioning range of motion, and even a little compromise in the sequence of movement will cause it considerable discomfort. Physical and emotional tension can be the cause, or may be contingent upon each other.

When great demands are made on the horse, as in high performance or racing, even the smallest changes and tensions will soon enough lead to poorer performance, and the horses then are, so to speak, "out of the race". But what about the other horses, whose 260 muscles perhaps do not have to work to such great demands but which still have to perform to a greater or lesser degree? How can we recognise, locate and rectify small problems before they cause damage that will later become evident in hand or under saddle, even when little is demanded of the horse?

The answers to these and other questions can be found described in the following chapters.

I am well aware that many experts are trying to help horses with related training, massage and pressure point systems, as well as through acupuncture and other methods, and some of their "new-found" (in reality, largely once-forgotten) methods, have achieved widespread interest. With this book, however, I would like to motivate you to try a method that has been successfully tried and tested by many horsemen and women all over the globe.

About my work

The pressure point system enables you to find and release tension in your horse. Don't get me wrong: educated specialists are there to help you with serious illnesses and you need them as much as your horse does. However, it often happens that you collect your horse, which for example has had a back problem, from the clinic, you pay the bill, and then you find the same problem returning after a short while.

Working with horses I hear stories like this on a daily basis. This has weighed heavily on my mind, because I am sure that the owners could have avoided or rectified the symptoms by following my simple programme. This treatment plan and its refined methods are a combined concept of physical and emotional components: a hotline to your horse.

First, I would like to explain the background. For years, my treatments all commenced with the same problem: "Chris, I have a problem with my horse and have tried everything. Could you please do something?" Even when the horse owner had no idea what I did, they trusted me because they had heard at second hand about me, and they probably felt they had nothing to lose. However, I could only help the horses in the short term, mainly because regular care was impossible due to distance. Although my previous patients went back to their owners recovered, as the owners did not know what I had done with their horses, they could not continue the therapy.

I received calls all the time with continuing questions and new problems, but because of the great distance between us I could not always look after my previous patients. I had dealt with all disciplines of horse sport and consequently developed a system of workshops that was in fact very general and easy to comprehend, and which could be used to understand and rectify the specific problems experienced by driving, riding and racehorses. The fruit of these thoughts is re-presented in this book, supplemented at the end with tips on gymnastic exercises for horses.

That I was on the right road was confirmed to me by amongst other things the questioning of hundreds of Canadian, American and Australian participants of the workshops. To what extent have they been successful after a course on the pressure point system and gymnastic exercises? Has that been reflected in a reduction in their veterinary expenses? Happily, everyone that continued to use this system was most satisfied with the unimpaired, willing performance of his or her horses. Their veterinary costs on average decreased from about $1500 to about

About my work

$500 per year. All the horses were uncomfortable before treatment due to tension and were restricted in their movement and performance.

It is clear that we should do whatever we can to assist in the health of our horses, because we are responsible for them. A lot of veterinarians have to live with the disappointment of knowing that some horses that have muscular or joint problems could have had it easier if their owner had only taken certain precautions. With the aid of this book, you will have the opportunity to save both yourself and your horse a lot of problems.

In the following chapters you will encounter a few expressions (doorbell, spider web etc.) that you may not necessarily associate with horses. They are however very useful in my work and will also soon make sense to you. I have travelled extensively, meeting committed people wanting to know more about my pressure point system, especially in the preventative field. I have enjoyed teaching them, but in the long run it was impossible to explain adequately the detailed, extensive and complicated medical context as well as the Latin terminology to everyone who came to me, with differing levels of previous knowledge. One day, as I tried to explain the structure and function of the long back muscle, the *lentissimo dorsi*, I shortened the lengthy explanation: I described the muscle simply as an elastic band that expands and contracts. Everyone understood immediately, so I started replacing more and more specialist medical terminology with more graphic terms and pictures that allowed freedom of association. This appeared to me to be so practical that I now feel completely comfortable with it.

Verbal analogies made it possible for me to teach technical experts as well as beginners in horse anatomy on the same workshop. Instead of having protracted discussions around the correct medical terminology, I prefer to point to the results of my work. Only these are of real interest to the horse and its owner. That is why you will find no detailed Latin terminology in this little book. If, however, you would like a more detailed physiological background, it would be best to consult a veterinary reference book on the subject.

After all my experience to date with this system to alleviate tension, I can virtually guarantee a positive result. That may sound presumptuous, but I believe in the system totally. For years, I saw again and again that literally everyone,

About my work

after one day at a lecture, was able to influence his or her horse's performance and behaviour in a positive way. The fact that most of my students were not burdened by deeper knowledge of muscle functions, but simply followed my advice on the eight point system, has been a decisive factor. The advice in this booklet is condensed and is intended to be as practical as possible, so that you can achieve the desired results very quickly. When I repeat myself at times, it serves both as a reminder of something and also means that you can reread individual chapters in isolation, without having to refer elsewhere in the book for explanation.

As your teacher I would like to impress upon you the importance of going through the basic steps, especially if you have had no experience with the pressure point system. Many of the students on my workshops were in the same situation.

> You can only gain nothing from the pressure point system if you do not use it!

Take this book with you to the stable, use it as a guide, look things up in it. As time goes by, you will master all the points. Don't be discouraged! The beginning is always difficult, but soon you will see your achievements and will be stimulated to learn more! Just like picking out feet or saddling your horse, the quick check and short treatment of problem zones will become part of your daily stable routine. These will enable both yourself and your horse to reap the benefits.

2. AROUND THE PRESSURE POINT SYSTEM

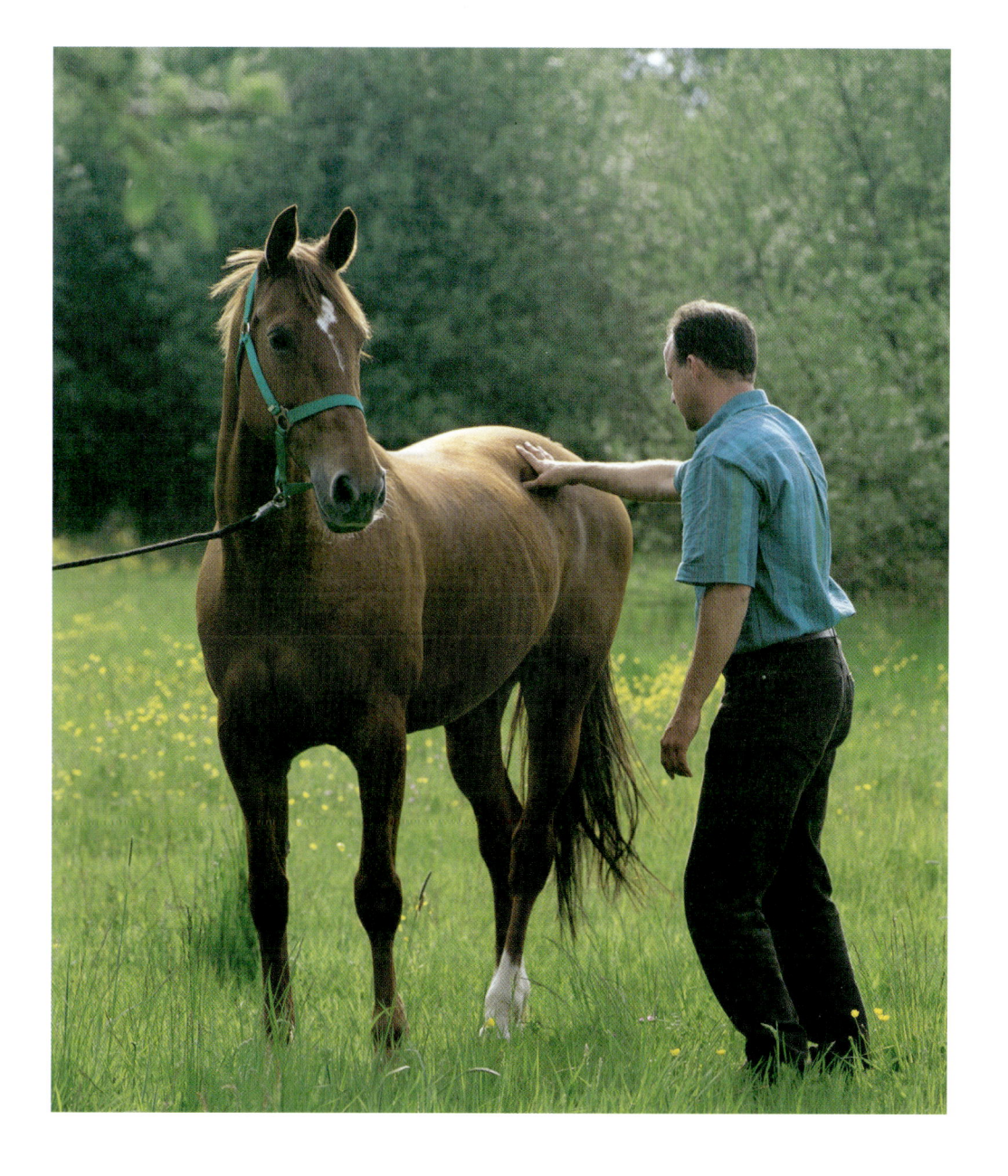

Around the pressure point system

The pressure point system (PPS) is nothing new. It has been used for more than 3,000 years. I have simply collected this ancient equine knowledge and condensed it. The system represented here, however, does not take all the muscles into consideration; rather it concentrates on the eight regions in the body of the horse that my work over the last twenty years has shown to me to be the areas that are most susceptible to tension.

I will highlight the extent to which a muscle with restricted function negatively influences surrounding tissue as well as other muscles.

Furthermore, I will show you that you need do no more than sensitise your fingers and eyes for tension and simply eliminate the build-up of problem zones. The eight points will help you initially to perform a complete examination on a regular basis, until the daily checks appear to be the most natural thing to do in the world.

Let us start from the assumption that as a beginner, starting your PPS training, you will track down only minor tightness. For the moment, that does not sound very satisfying, but in a few weeks you will accumulate sufficient practical knowledge that your technique improves in leaps and bounds. This is the secret of PPS: you simply do it, and before you know, you will be sharing your experiences with other horsemen and women.

> The most important point in PPS is that we go direct to the cause of many problems, rather than simply dealing with the symptoms.

2.1. MUSCLES: WHERE TENSION STARTS

Roughly 260 muscles keep your horse going, by contracting and then pulling bones in the direction of the contraction. Bones are connected to muscles with tendons, and every muscle has a partner that works with it. The tightening of one muscle will only be successful when its partner, working in the opposite direction, is completely relaxed and fully extended.

In this phase of total relaxation the muscle gets refuelled with blood and oxygen, the fuel it uses to contract; at the same time it removes waste products (carbon dioxide and lactic acid) that build up in the muscle.

To ensure that the animal can move freely, all these aspects have to work together effortlessly.

Around the pressure point system

Pressure, bumps, injury or illness can all cause a muscle to be "scared" into contraction. The muscle may only tense up to a certain extent, and the blood flow is compromised at this point.

Other muscle fibres have to take over the work from their crippled colleagues, then they in turn become overtaxed – the tension builds up. The tendons also are affected by this downward spiral and can become entwined in the whole event.

Shown in Figure 1 is the muscle with the tendon that performs with it. Both sides are included in the tautness, so where, if I may ask, is the onset of tension? At the muscle or at the tendon? My answer is: at the tendon.

In Figure 2 you can see it more precisely: the muscle and its tension work in close proximity to each other.

The small lines in Figure 2 indicate thousands of hairline fibres that attach to the end of the tendon and extend into the body of the muscle. The green point is a location where collection of tissue fluid takes place, called oedema. Oedema has various functions; it will for example act as a "cleaner" to get rid of all the old and dead cells.

Now this is the question: how does oedema get into the tendon?

When any kind of tissue is damaged, whether due to illness, operation, over-exertion or other reasons, there will be a collection of fluid in the tissue. Ordinarily that would not be too bad, for under normal circumstances it would disappe-

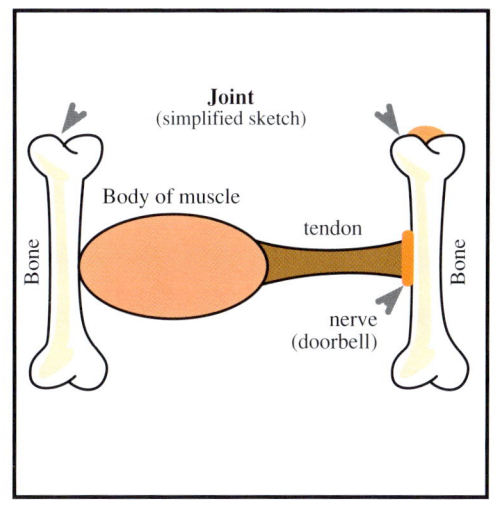

1: Simplified sketch of the body of a muscle, connected to the bone via a tendon bone, joint (taken apart), body of muscle, tendon (doorbell)

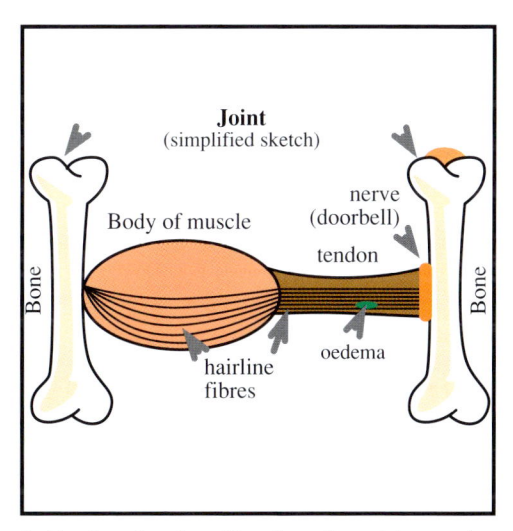

2: Muscle and tendon with oedema. Bone, joint, muscle, nerve, hairline fibres, oedema

Around the pressure point system

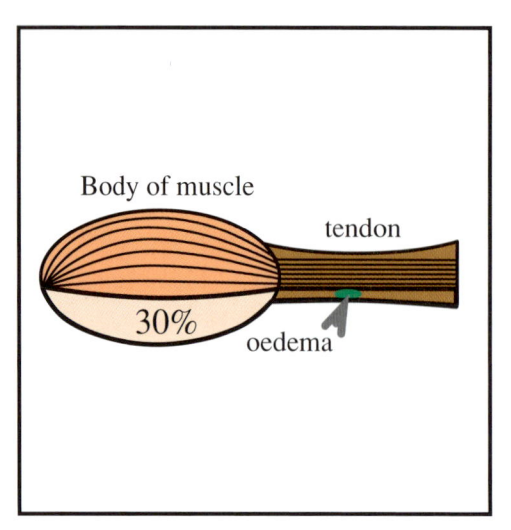

3: Shortened fibres caused by oedema. At 30% it influences the fibres and is visible

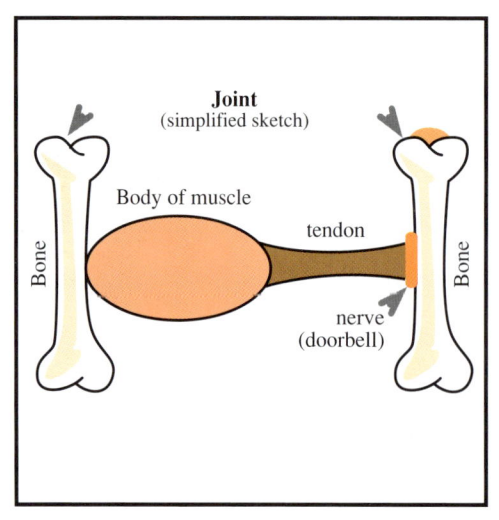

4: Muscle, tendon, nerve: between the bone and the tendon lies the nerve. With tension within the muscle-tendon unit, any pressure will ring the doorbell

ar by itself, especially through movement. When a horse has little or no possibility of movement, either because of a condition of illness or long periods of standing still, the oedema will harden within about four months.

As long as the oedema stays small and no other tissue becomes seized, you will in all probability find no impairment to your horse's performance or well-being. It is only when about 30 per cent of the tissue gets blocked that you will notice a definite change in behaviour. This manifests itself for example by being ticklish when being groomed, resistance to bending or to holding an outline, diminishing performance, inadequate straightness or collection, increased shying, and so on. The blame should not be attributed to "mood swings", but rather the distress of the painful, ever-growing tension that has not been observed by you.

The question now is: when did these difficulties commence? Was it in the moment that you noticed it, or rather weeks, months or even years before?

What happens when approximately 30 per cent of a tendon is blocked with oedema?

The fine tendon tissue is connected to the muscle fibre, which means that approximately 30 per cent of the body of the muscle is also involved. The blood flow is restricted, the muscle does not function perfectly, it loses much of its flexibility and in doing so weakens the muscle-tendon unit (Figure 3).

Around the pressure point system

Between the tendon and the bone lies a nerve that I would simply refer to as "the doorbell". This terminology will help, if you have no previous knowledge of anatomy or any diagrams of muscles, to detect tension in the horse. This way both laymen and experts can be equally effective.

I would like you to do a little experiment that will help make the rest of this book easier to understand: relax your hand (Figure 5) and push down, as with a doorbell, onto the tendons. You will probably not notice much.

Now make a fist (Figure 6; you are now simulating tension) and press down again. When firm pressure is exerted on a specific point, you will quickly experience a slight pain: "the doorbell will ring".

The same thing happens when oedema gets trapped in a tendon. To all intents and purposes this "bell" rings regularly when oedema is present in a tendon, and you can be assured that it will start to ring with a mere 5 per cent of oedema present.

I have already mentioned (Figure 3) that approximately 30 per cent oedema in the tendon can be seen by the untrained eye once the horse starts to move. The difference is now that you realise this; with the help of the "doorbell", you are in a position to identify even minute tightness.

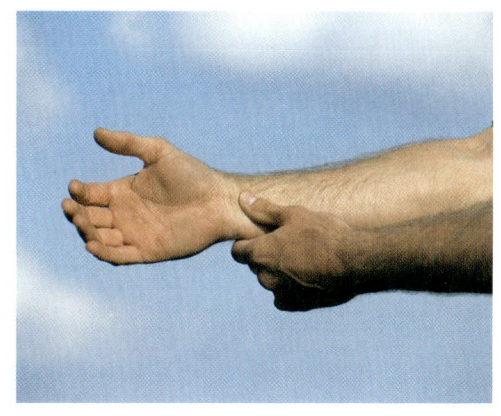

5: Hold your hand relaxed in front of you, push on the tendons: no pain is felt.

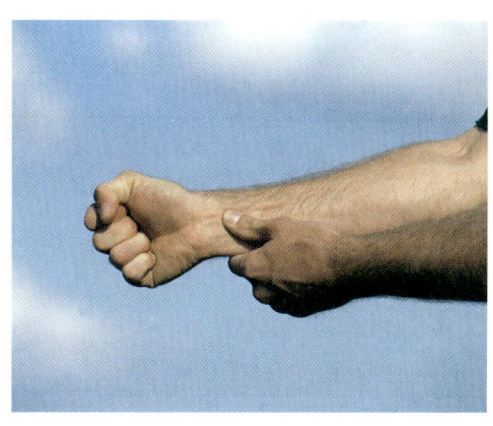

6: Make a fist. Now you simulate tension in the fibres. Push on the tendons. You will soon notice that it hurts; this is the nerve, the "doorbell" that points to the tension. With the help of this tendon connection you can also find tension in horses.

In other words, by using PPS you will locate invisible tension BEFORE it has a chance to harm your horse. Why should you wait for the problem to turn into an obvious predicament? By using the "doorbell" you can immediately find and eliminate it.

2.2. ELIMINATING TENSION IN MUSCLES

When you see a drawing of a horse's muscles, you can distinguish between hundreds of small, medium and large sections. I shall not confuse you with unnecessary detail, but restrict the PPS to using only eight regions. With the concept of the "doorbell" you can locate and remove tension in the muscles without any fuss or detailed knowledge of names and their locations.

Right at the beginning of our training I would like to give you a small functional introduction to PPS, that will illustrate the additional tasks and later be explained in greater detail when you learn about region 4. Believe me, learning to find tightness in muscles could not be easier.

The most difficult task for me is to convince you to actually go and try it! With this book to hand, get on the way to your four-legged friend and have a go at the following procedures. When you have settled yourself in a little corner to read, let us do the first manoeuvres together, so that you may master the technique as soon as possible in the interest of your horse.

Right, all being well, you are now standing next to your horse. Have a good

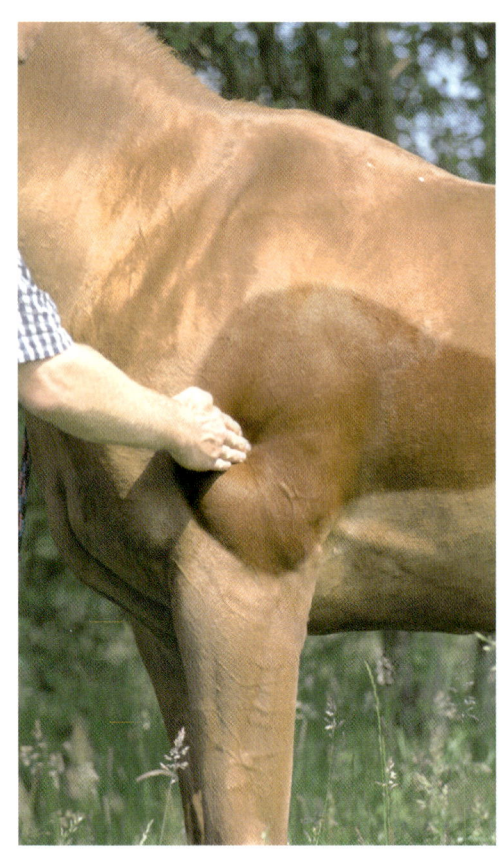

7: Test inside the marked area for tension

look at Figure 7. This region is very suitable for demonstrating to horse owners how easy it is to detect any slight tautness that can be cleared away by anybody. Now it is your turn!

> All circular movements should be carried out in an anticlockwise direction.

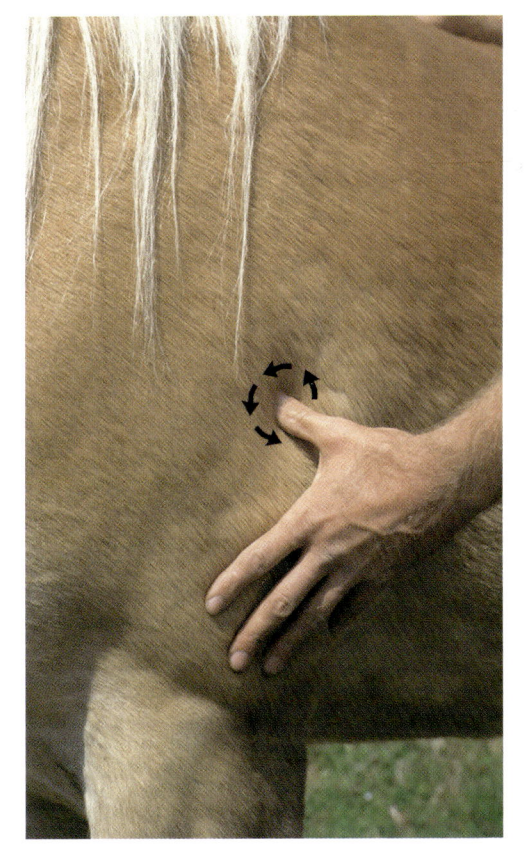

8: Move your thumb in an anticlockwise direction where you have found tightness. Use about the same amount of pressure as in our test in Fig. 6

2.3. FINGERTIPS AND MORE

For the removal of oedema, you will often use a circular pressure technique. In Figure 8 you can see a thumb pressing down, while at the same time moving in a circular direction. Imagine how you can use that to dispel fluid build-up and stimulate the tendon. It is important to remember how hard you had to push down on your wrist. Feel free to carry out the experiment in Figure 6 again.

In the following chapters I will frequently refer back to that, so that you can estimate the amount of pressure needed on your horse.

I would like to explain in a very elementary way what influence the pressure has.

The stimulation of the tendon arouses the brain to distribute substances that promote the flow of blood to the inflamed area within approximately 10 minutes. You will detect this through the warming up of the area.

All treated surfaces will experience this increased circulation for hours after manipulation. This improved blood flow then assists the neighbouring muscles to be more flexible for approximately three hours afterwards.

More detailed information can be found in medical textbooks.

Around the pressure point system

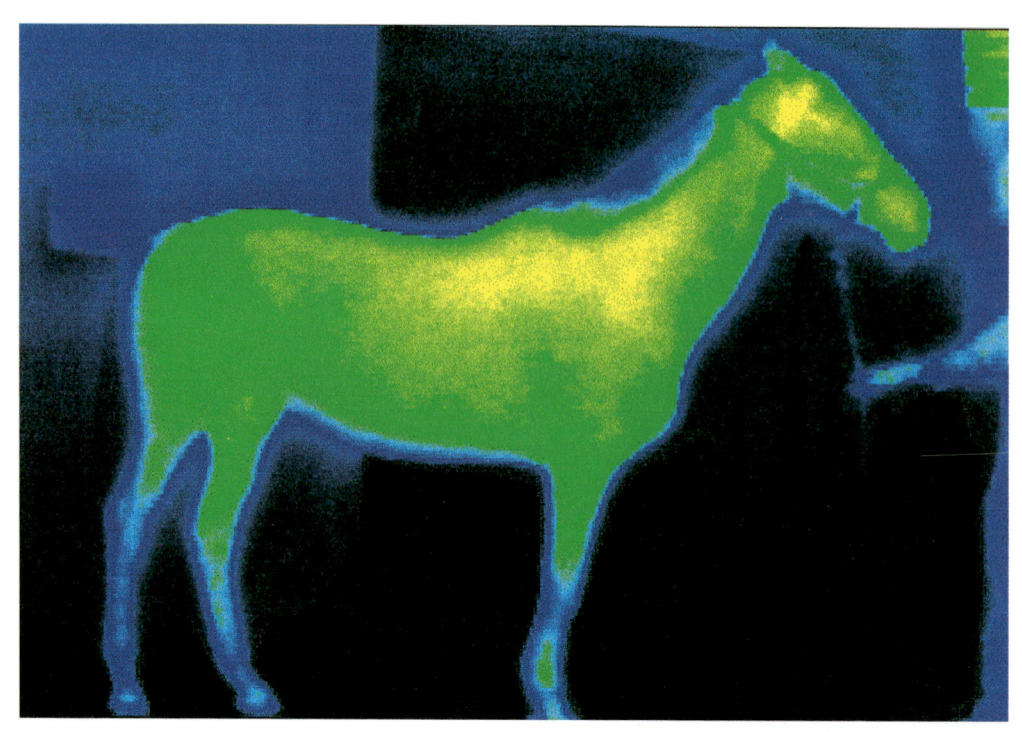

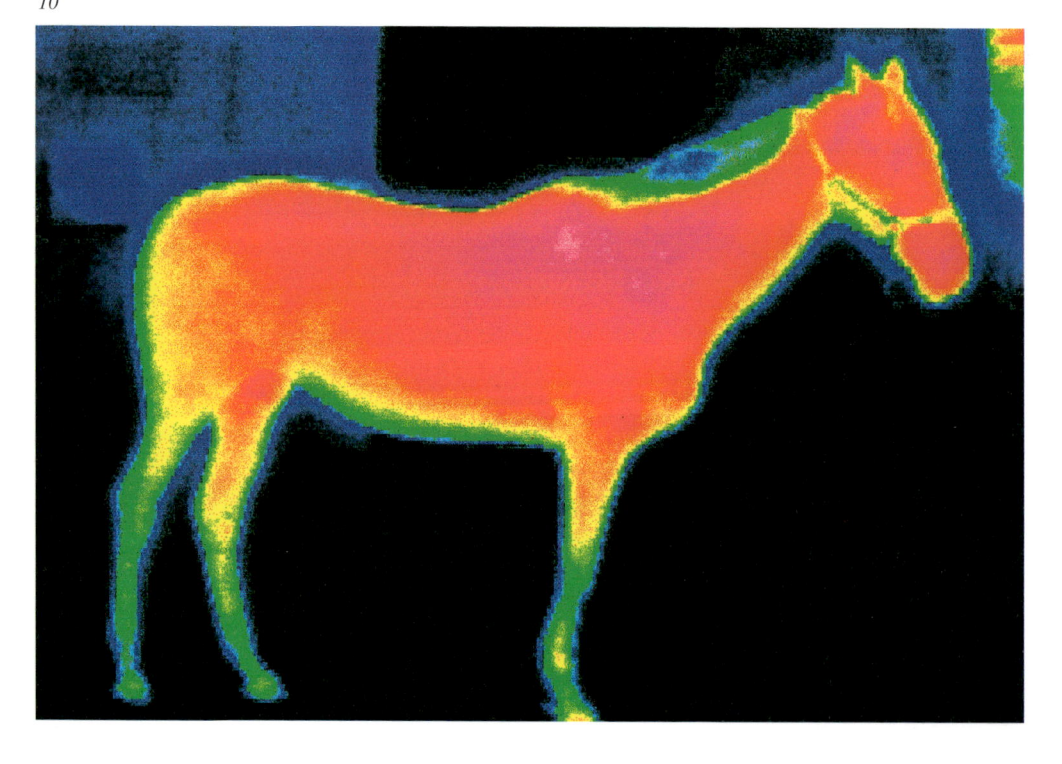

9
10

2.4. SAFETY PRECAUTIONS

Please take this advice seriously, for occasionally our four-legged patients experience agony before relief, and can behave in an unpredictable, even forceful way initially. This kind of response will soon peter out as the therapy starts to be effective.

- *Do not work for longer than five minutes in any region. Normally one or two minutes will be sufficient in your regular examinations.*
When starting PPS, when the old tensions may be deep-seated, it is better to repeat the treatment frequently.
- *Do not massage when a horse has a high temperature or fever, inflammation, heart problems or eczema.*
- *Use a head collar with a lead rein.*
- *Under no circumstances should you work in the horse's stable or in any other confined space.*
- *Horses can react in an unpredictable way to long-term suffering. Some areas should be concentrated on in your treatment.*
- *At first the pressure can be uncomfortable for the horse (this will dissipate) but he may under no circumstances be startled by it.*
- *Assuming the horse dodges and moves away, I would recommend you get a helper on the other side of the horse.*
- *All small animals (cats, dogs) as well as obstacles (buckets etc.) should be removed while treating a horse, to stop you from tripping over them in the event of having to make a hasty exit.*

9/10: To convince you right from the beginning that PPS is good for blood flow, infra-red pictures show a horse before (9) and after (10) treatment.
The tension in this horse caused serious impediment to the blood flow. Red and yellow colours show the spontaneous warmth generated with the PPS.
The thermographic expert Wilfrid Schlosser provided these pictures.

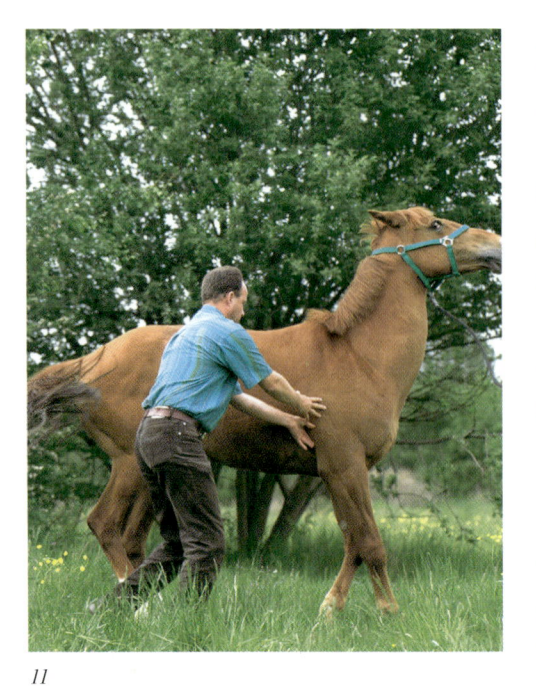

Around the pressure point system

2.5. FEEL THE DIFFERENCE!

Press down firmly on your horse at the point shown in Figure 8. Don't be afraid that you will injure your horse!

Just consider how loutish they occasionally are in the paddock, how they bite and kick at each other. I assure you,

11/12: This horse is in severe pain.
She swishes her tail, runs around and rears (Fig.12) in her efforts to get away from the pain. Please take extra care when treating your horse if you are not yet sure how severe the pain is.
Before being treated, the chestnut mare had been serenely quiet, but with no more than light poking exploded.
The new owner looked on in horror.
However, after the treatment, the mare was ready for a new life, free of pain…

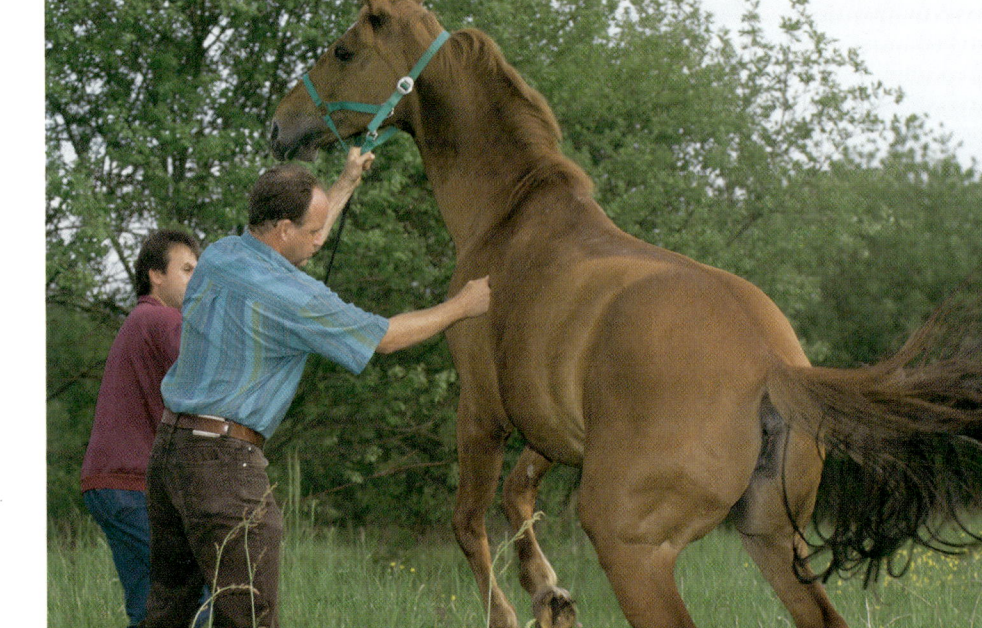

11

12

Around the pressure point system

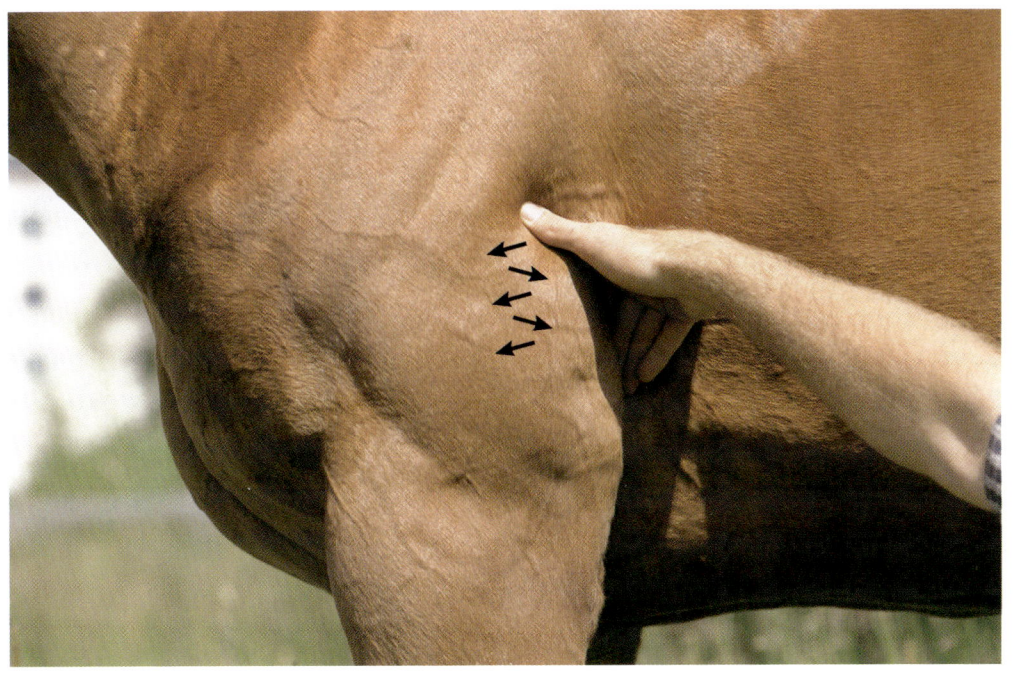

13: When you find tension in this region, it is time to remove it. Look for the body of a muscle, about 3cm across. Move the fingers to and fro towards the bottom of the muscle. There you will find the tendon. Massage with circular movements for a few minutes, and then go back to the area where you originally found the tension. Is there a small improvement? Well done!

your fingers can do no damage. So go for it – press down on the area shown in Figure 8. If you are reading this book because your horse has some tightness, then I am sure you will generate some flinches to a greater or lesser degree.

The bell is ringing – there is resident tension. Otherwise just poke purposefully around the location inside this region. This poking should be done so firmly that your fingertips actually spring back from the horse's body.

Pay attention to where and how strongly the bell rings, but it does not always have to be as violent as in Figures 11 and 12. Does your horse twitch its skin? Does he strike with his head or tail? Do these same reactions occur while you are grooming your horse?

Resume the pressure, even when the reactions are at a minimum, for I would like you to distinguish the different strengths of the pressure you use.

My intention now is that you should notice some small improvement, even when this is the first time you are using PPS. Corresponding to Figures 11 and 12, you have perceived where the ten-

Around the pressure point system

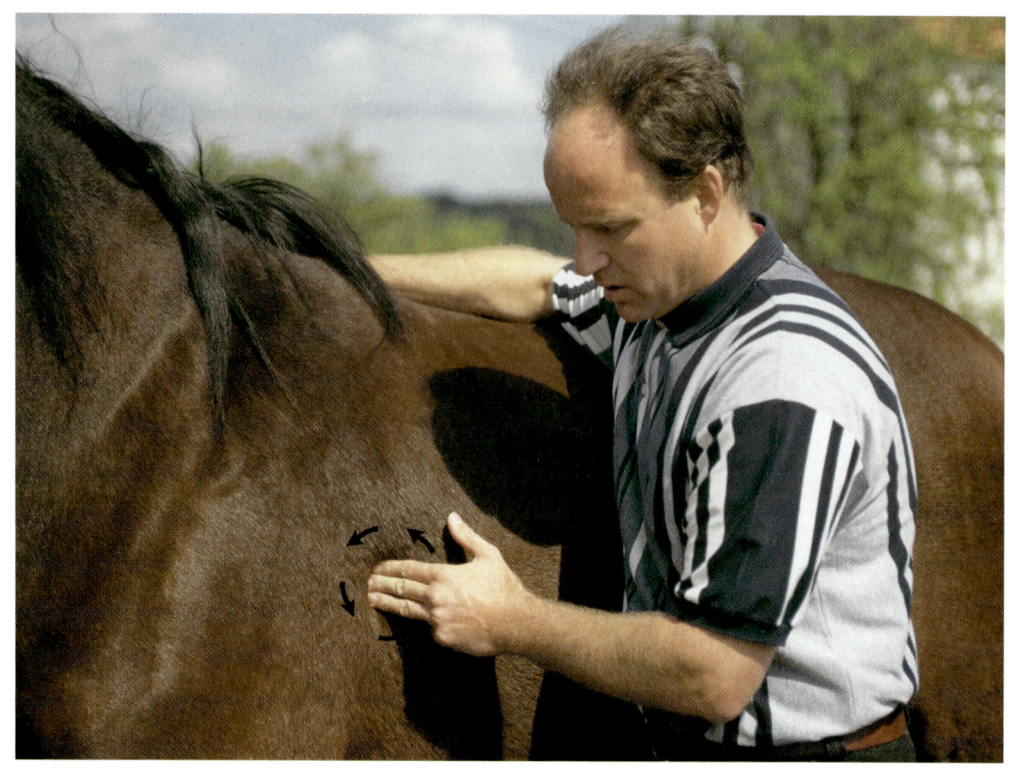

14: The fingertip technique supplements the thumb technique and is frequently used. For maximum effect it is better to use the three middle fingers, again in an anticlockwise direction. This is useful when your thumbs are tired.

sion exists, because the doorbell addressed the twitching.

Now put your thumb on the area in Figure 13. Press down firmly and maintain the pressure, then rub backwards and forwards. In doing this you will feel the body of a muscle (about the size of a thumb) under the skin. Good! Move your thumb again; manoeuvre it in all directions, also up and down across the small body of the muscle. Eventually you will detect that this muscle is getting softer and moreover smaller, until you can hardly feel it any more. Perform the circular fingertip technique once more over the whole section (Figure 14).

What I would like most is to be able to stand next to you, so that I could personally observe your progress, but even if it takes a little longer by yourself, you will come to a positive conclusion. You will just have to trust the bell that will show you if there is any tension.

When the tension you have found cannot be pushed away, the bell will go on ringing.

Around the pressure point system

> Do you recall how violently your horse responded and in which area it was when you examined your horse a few minutes ago for the first time with the finger pressure? When you meticulously followed my instructions, found a doorbell and treated the tautness accordingly, then the response from your horse after ten minutes should have subsided to a tiny fraction of the initial reaction. Is that enough? YES, because every time that you employ PPS, the result will be improved upon.

Let us just recollect everything so far:

You can also compare the reaction you get with the other side that has not been treated, which will respond by being "ticklish" while the side that has been treated with PPS will only provoke a slight reaction. If you miss out on a few areas of tension – no problem! Simply attempt it again (maybe on another horse with more pronounced problems) in the manner described and eventually you can be sure to make a strike. Do not give up hope! Practice with PPS definitely makes perfect, and a little bit of patience goes a long way. Hopefully, I am now able to congratulate you, for you have just become proficient in finding tension in muscles and eliminating it. You will ask in complete amazement: "Is it that easy?" Can so little effort deliver such a result? CERTAINLY! It really is that simple, but in the meanwhile you have recognised it for yourself. You should approach the other aspects in much the same way. The most important concept for a start is that you know: I can do this!

Let us now, being newly motivated, examine more theory and discuss why a single tensed-up muscle can actually affect the whole integrated sequence of the horse's movement.

3. JUST ONE SINGLE TENSED-UP MUSCLE, BUT…

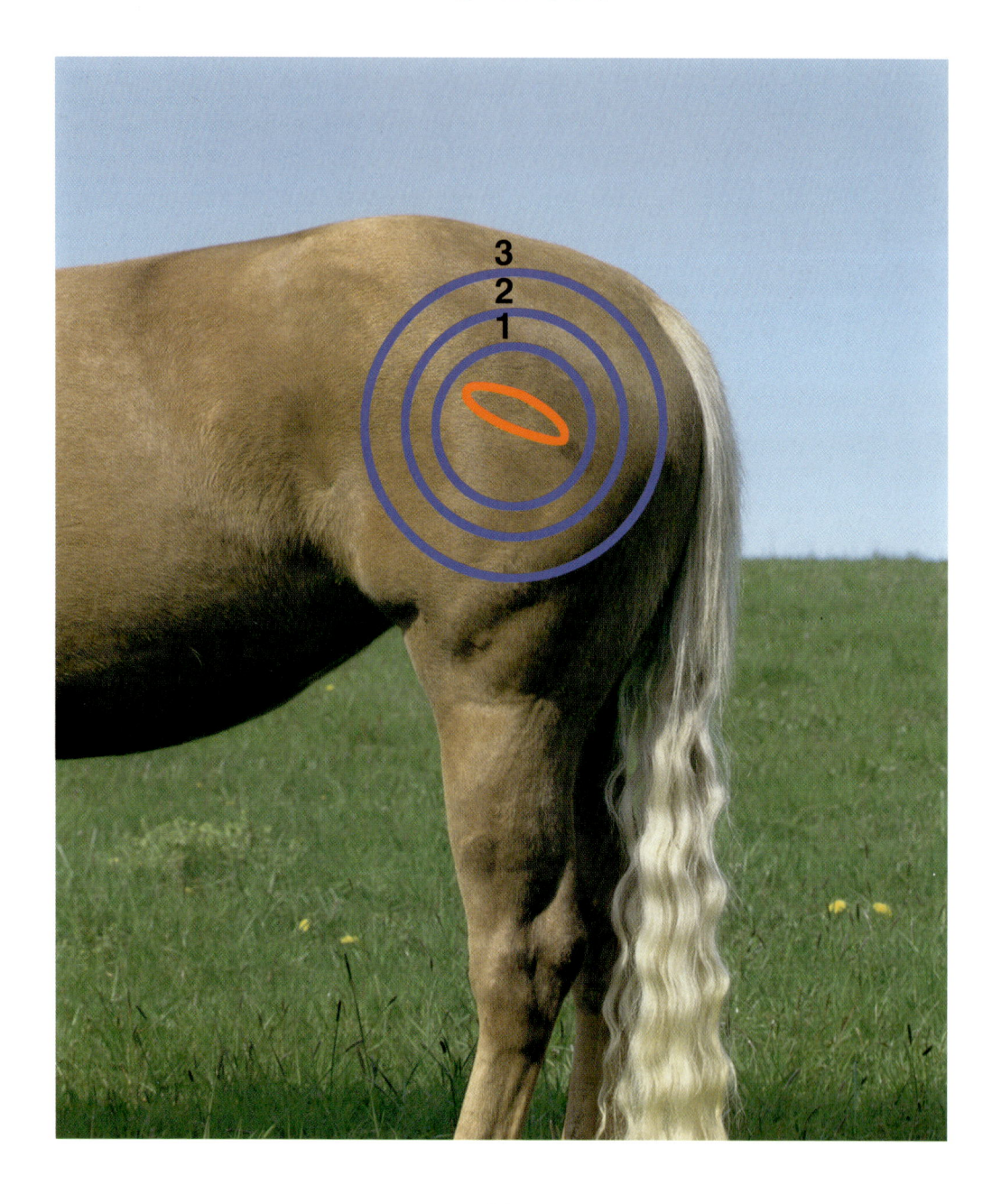

The entire muscular system of any animal is interwoven like a spider's web. One single tensed-up muscle will therefore affect all the other healthy muscles.

The red section in Figure 15 denotes a tensed-up muscle. As we have observed before, a muscle-tendon combination shortens when oedema is stuck in the tissue, which means the tendon and muscle fibres that are connected with each other are now bonded together and have lost a considerable amount of their elasticity.

The following happens: when the muscle fibres in the red section can no longer perform at 100 per cent, they ask their neighbours if they can be of any assistance. In other words the red muscle turns to blue muscle group 1 for moral support. Blue muscle group 1 cooperates, but now has a lot more work to do, so asks support from blue muscle group 2. After a while, blue muscle group 2 now starts to suffer and begs support from blue muscle group 3 etc. In this way all the muscle groups surrounding the taut muscle will gradually suffer.

15: The red marked area is a taut muscle. The loss of movement must be compensated for by the neighbouring muscles in blue group 1, that is then helped by group 2, then group 3 and so on. A little bit of tension is then carried over into a much bigger area.

The originally trivial problem has become a big problem. When the right hindquarter is only modestly fit for use, the impairment will at some time or other have an effect on the left shoulder or forehand. Why does that happen? All movements need a diagonal support, and in this way, the diagonal counterpart of the tensed-up hindquarter will try and compensate for the shortage of power, so that a balanced flow of movement, in harmony with the other diagonal, is guaranteed.

Right in the middle of all this is the big back muscle, the "elastic band".

3.1. THE ELASTIC BAND

There is a remarkably big muscle (Longissimus dorsi, Figure 16) across the back of the horse that I would like to describe as a type of elastic band. It connects and coordinates the sequence of movements between the forehand and the hindquarters. In the illustration, the muscles of the right forehand (region 1) and the right hindquarters are under strain. Please observe the direction in which the forces work and the arrows move (1 = forwards, 2 = backwards).

The "elastic band" tries, even while standing, to recoil to its original position,

Just one single tensed-up muscle, but...

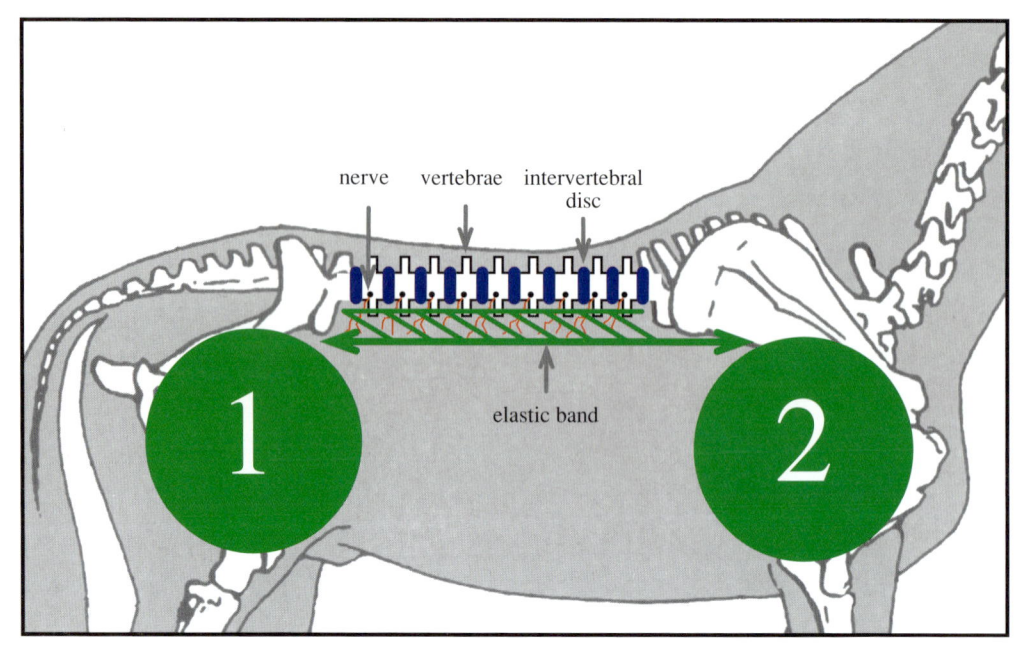

16: The big back muscle of the horse, the Longissimus dorsi (simplified) is called the elastic band in this book. Depending on the movement, it stretches and goes back into position. From an anatomical viewpoint any tension between the forehand and hindquarters has a negative influence.

but that cannot be done when one of its muscle-tendon units is shortened because it has been strained. It does not make any difference whether the horse moves or stands: the elastic band is always taut.

Back problems are the cause of suffering in a lot of horses. In sport, a back problem often means the beginning of the end. Do not believe that you can escape the problem by using gel pads or thick numnahs. That is just pulling wool over your eyes; your horse will not be pleased with that. Most horses suffer especially in the back area from ill-fitting saddles (that goes for most of us), insufficient knowledge of riding, or classical, never-relieved stiffness.

3.2. THE SPINAL COLUMN

The spinal column is a fantastic arrangement of nature with really complicated functions, but the problems that arise there can easily be explained. An elastic band that is always rigid and which over a period of years, presses on the spinal column, has a lot to do with it as far as I am concerned. Between the vertebrae, there are intervertebral discs

Just one single tensed-up muscle, but...

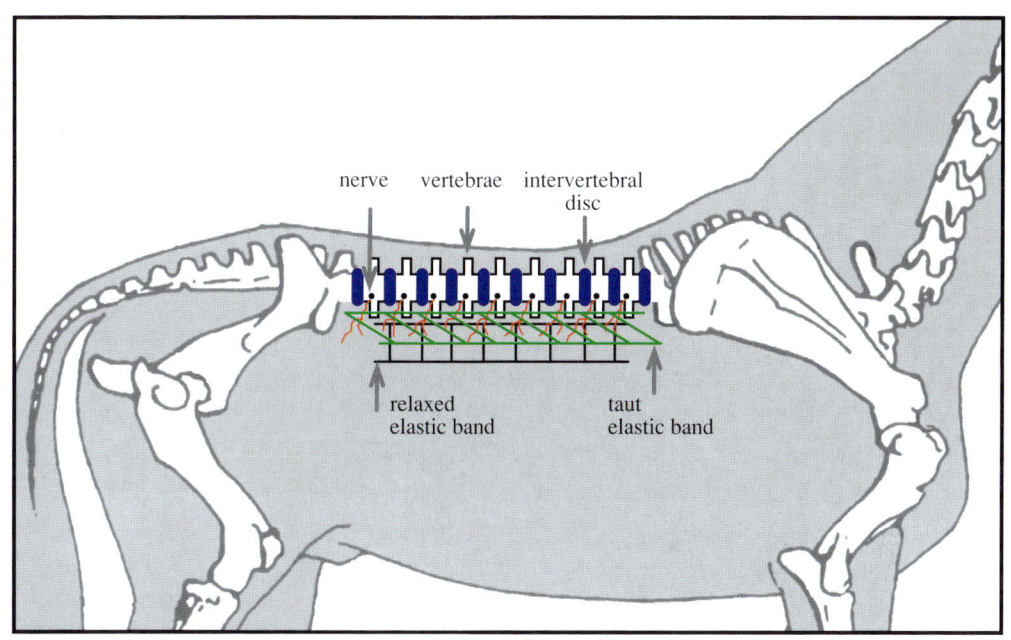

17: There are intervertebral discs and nerves between the vertebrae. When the elastic band is tight, the vertebrae and the discs are pressed together, eventually pinching the nerves.

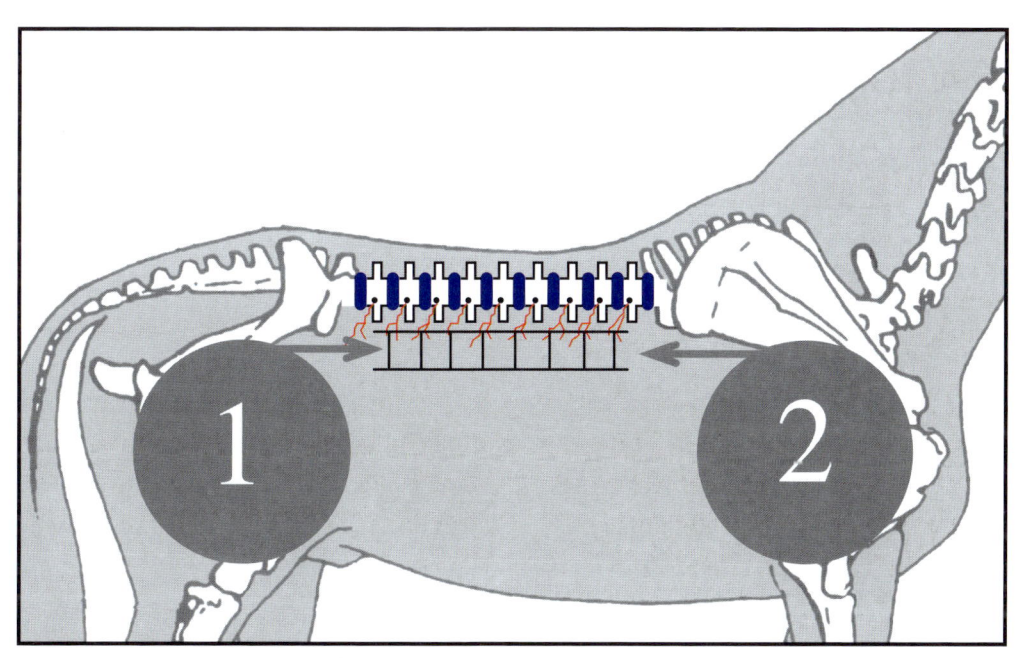

18: After treatment with PPS, the elastic band can relax due to the loosened regions at 1 and 2. There is enough space between the muscle and the vertebrae for free movement.

that are filled with a glutinous liquid. In the long run, not even the strongest discs can withstand the continuous pressure, and little by little, these will become constricted and start to atrophy.

In order for the discs to take up some liquid, they need to be relatively free in movement, but as long as the forehand or hindquarters of the horse are under tension, this cannot happen. The taut elastic band caused by the shortened muscle-tendon unit burdens the vertebrae and jams the discs even more.

With such tightness, the vertebrae suffer even when the horse is resting, just as the elastic band is permanently under strain and pressure.

In a stiff horse the elastic band will constrict the vertebrae and press the discs together. In severe cases, the nerves will also become trapped. See red marked nerves in Figure 17.

In the following chapters, I will explain how you can make use of this sensitive area of the back to test in general for tension in a horse. In order for the vertebrae to perform perfectly, there must be no pressure on them. The discs have to be able to move freely; otherwise they will atrophy and restrict the blood flow, even damaging the nerves.

This burden can only be lifted from the back when the elastic band is relaxed. In Figure 18 you will see the blue regions 1 and 2 after treatment with PPS. It is very important that the arrows now point to each other. The vertebrae can consequently relax with the elastic band; the discs can absorb liquid and become regenerated. Into the bargain, the vertebrae can move away from each other again and the pressure on the nerves will ease off.

You can come to your own conclusion when you think about the phenomenon of kissing spines, where the vertebrae of the back knock together, causing considerable obstruction and enormous discomfort in the horse. So long as the vertebrae or discs are not yet permanently damaged or have some chronic condition, I have to say that I have had a 100 per cent success rate when using PPS on horses with kissing spines. They can become fit and healthy once again and with thoughtful training, where the muscles get built up properly, they can overcome all their problems.

When you see to it that the elastic band is relaxed again, then the vertebrae will no longer jolt together. The vertebrae, like the rest of the skeleton, do not have a life of their own, but are passive components of the system of movement. The bones of the skeleton are entirely dependent on the muscles for holding them in the correct positions.

Just one single tensed-up muscle, but...

3.3. JOINT DAMAGE

You have received some insight into the correlation between tension and health associated with joint problems. However, my experience and assumptions extend further, and I would like to describe the explanations I have found, amongst others, for problems in the joints.

In Figure 19 you see the hindquarter with the relevant muscles portrayed as a spider's web. The blue line illustrates the muscle-tendon units that reach down to the hoof of the horse.

19: The muscle groups are connected like a spider's web. The blue line points to the group of muscles, tendons and nerves of the hind leg. Tension can have a negative influence on the joints, for example the hock.

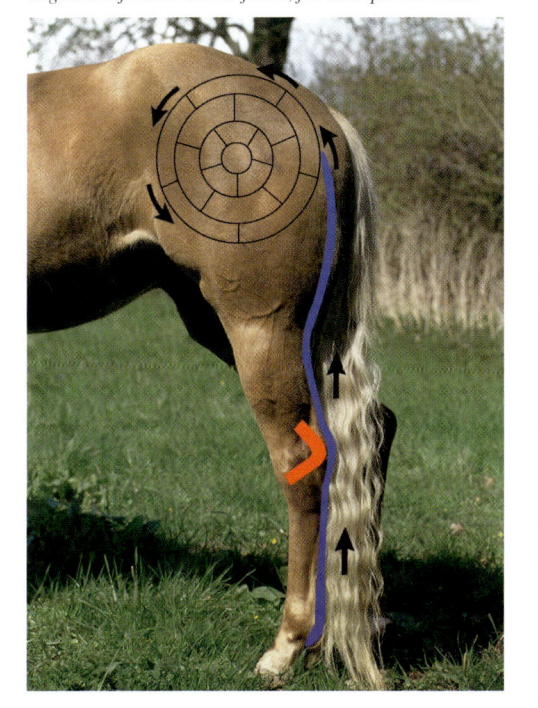

The hock repeatedly suffers when you get tension within the spider's web.

Do you recollect? When a muscle is taut, it shortens and then pulls even healthy muscles into its direction, shown here by the path of the arrows on the blue line, bearing along to the spider's web.

The continual tug on the tight muscle-tendon unit in the hindquarter keeps the joints in the leg under strain, and so aggravating the condition on a daily basis.

Maybe your horse already had problems in this area, but it is certainly possible that tension can account for lameness or difficulty in this joint, especially if there is no trauma due to any definite and unusual way of moving or known injury. (I have noticed this in hundreds of horses I have treated.) If the cause of the problem is just tension, you will find after treatment of the strained muscle parts that your horse will begin to experience positive regeneration. When the pull on that joint disappears, it is of major importance to methodically rebuild the relaxed muscle.

> The relieving of tense muscles alone is not enough. Strong, healthy muscles participate to support the joints in their job. You must also pay attention to the rebuilding of muscles.

4. PHYSICAL RELAXATION: THE PRESSURE POINT SYSTEM (PPS)

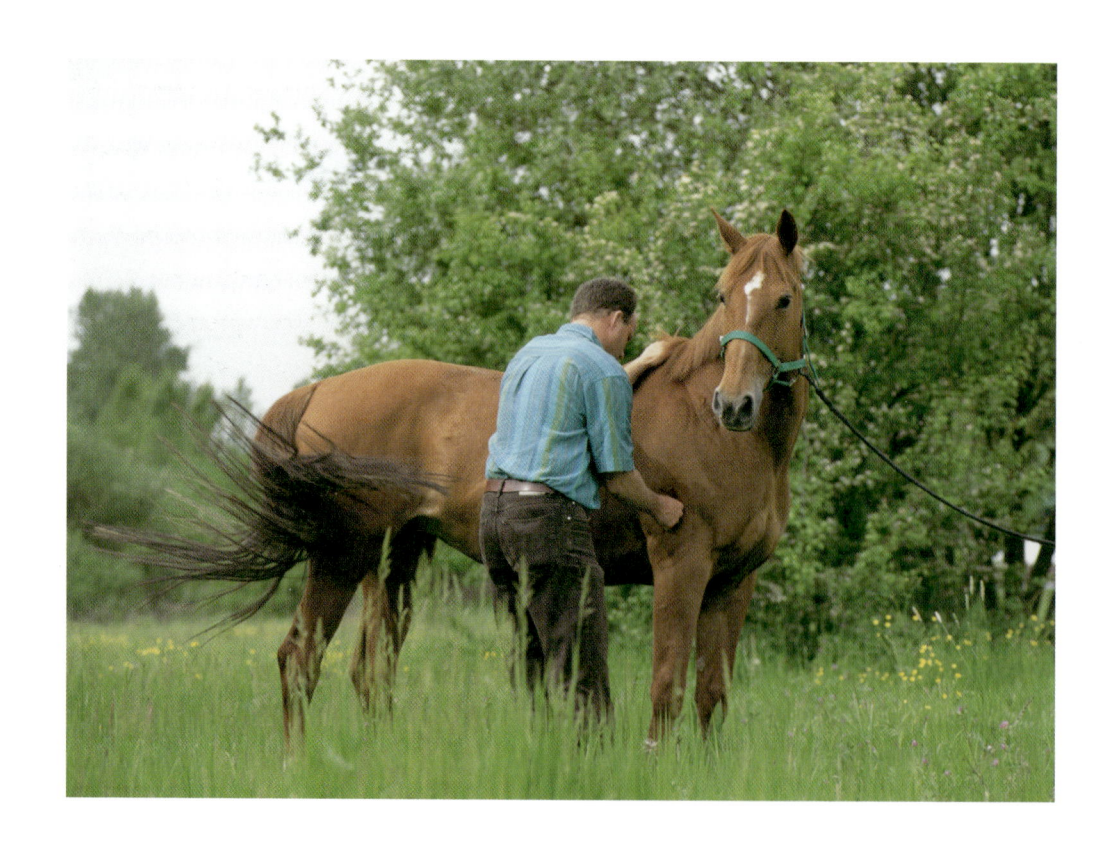

Physical relaxation: the pressure point system

You have now ascertained, as illustrated by practical implementation of the pressure point system, that it is perfectly straightforward. As with all things new, you will find that by applying it and doing so repeatedly, your technique will improve.

I am drawing on the pool of knowledge that horsemen and women have been using for over 3,000 years, and I see the principle of this book as being the connection that I am making between you as the owner of a horse and the pressure point system.

I have simplified and concentrated it into eight areas to work on. These eight areas would, however, not be sufficient when a qualified physiotherapist treated a profoundly tensed-up horse. For your own personal use, the system should prove quite satisfactory, as countless numbers of people from my courses have already found. I am deliberately omitting complex, multifaceted problems that only an experienced therapist should tackle, and am concentrating on the areas that will concern you the most.

Next time you are considering whether or not you need to call a therapist to see your horse, do not be too concerned. It may not be possible for you to eliminate all the tension by using PPS, but you will definitely be able to relieve some of it. The condition of your horse will most certainly not deteriorate. Rather 1 per cent success than none at all. It makes no difference whether you are a competing rider or just have fun hacking out: if your horse happens to have any tension somewhere, you will be better able to identify and eliminate it.

> Once you have mastered the pressure point system, I would like to invite you to share your experiences with other friends of horses. That way you will not only gain more confidence, but you will ensure that more horses are sound in the future.

The eight regions are the areas which, when in motion, are burdened the most in relation to other areas of the horse´s body. Figure 20 shows these areas. After we have successfully completed our first practical training session together, you may doubt me when I say that you legitimately know enough to proceed to the other regions. But I mean that in earnest! You know how to make the bell ring, and how to relieve or eradicate the tension. The only additional knowledge you require now is a few extra pressure techniques as well as some insight to the precise location of the zones of stress.

Physical relaxation: the pressure point system

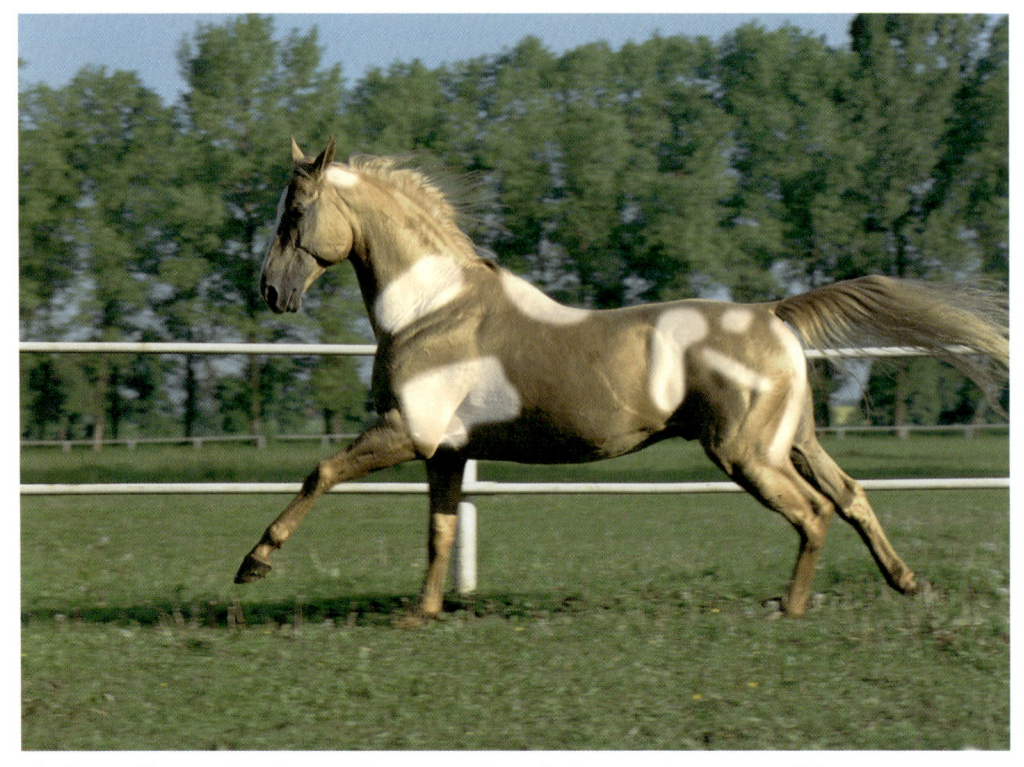

20: Illustrated here are the eight regions for treatment. Naturally there are other areas as well, but experience has taught me that these eight are where most problems occur, which can be treated by almost everybody.

I know from the workshops I run that some of you are frightened by the sometimes violent reactions of your horses. Even when you cause, in the subsequent period of time, a lot more discomfort, these circumstances are justified by the results that occur later, namely a considerable improvement in your horse's well-being.

I still find it astonishing how horses react to PPS. During the first treatment, where everything is still new and out-of-the-ordinary, they tend to be uneasy. That changes abruptly when the stimulation of the tendons triggers the release of positive substances that give the horse the feeling of total relaxation (just think how you feel after a good massage). This state of affairs manifests itself after approximately ten minutes. A good many horses actually fall asleep.

Some of them experience such a feeling of well-being with the therapy, that in an endeavour to get more pressure they push with all their might against the fingers and will even give the therapist (in this case it is you) an energetic prod with the head to indicate the region they

Physical relaxation: the pressure point system

> The horse will always tell you with its body language whether you are in the right position. Keep your eyes peeled during treatments: Does the horse breathe deeply? Is he relaxing? Does he close his eyes? Is he lowering his head? Are the ears turning to the side? Is the horse moving the treated body part in the direction of the therapist? Those are the unmistakable signs that the horse is feeling satisfied.
>
> Butting with the head, flicking the tail, twitching of the skin, restless stepping this and that way, yes, even nipping and kicking can be an indication of suffering when you are treating profoundly strained body parts. As soon as the circulation has been improved and the tension is starting to clear away, it is quite possible that after the first session of treatment the horse will no longer behave badly.

behaviour, before I commence work with the pressure point therapy. The explanation is fundamental: just think to what extent stress at work can involve your own muscles, for example, in your neck and shoulders.

Tension headaches and back pain are the end product of that stress. The same eventually applies to your horse. Stress and tension can easily extend over his whole body when he is not in emotional equilibrium, or is feeling unwell.

> The emotional stimulus of stress is frequently terribly underestimated. It is generally much less complicated to solve muscular tension when a horse is emotionally at ease.

would like you to massage next. That is a tremendous feeling!

Please keep in mind that some horses have never been able to relax in their whole lives, living as they do in noisy and bustling yards. In my courses or treatments, I will in general be first and foremost concerned with the mind, meaning problems with the psyche and

In the following chapters, I do not wish to illustrate the objective of each of the treated muscles, but I would like you to concentrate on the addressed muscles on both sides of the body. It is not important on which side you commence; what is essential is that you work through all the points from 1 to 8 before you move to the other side. The described locations can vary in the individual anatomy of the horse, depending on its breed, training and muscular development.

Physical relaxation: the pressure point system

4.1. THE FIRST TEST

The only things you need in order to go in search of tension are two fingers or both thumbs. Pass your fingers slowly along, next to the vertebrae on the back, and in fact, from the back towards the front. Remember the illustration of vertebrae in Figure 17?

When a horse has tautness in this area of the elastic band, regardless of how tight it is, the nerves will be irritated by your fingers running along the back, and you will see a typical evasive reaction, frequently interpreted as being ticklish or sensitive.

The back is either as hard as a board or drops down, seemingly flinching from the discomfort. A lot of horses also butt with the head or flick their tails.

Press and pass your fingers rapidly along the back in the direction indicated by the blue line in Figure 21 to examine it. If there is no reaction, repeat the action, with a little more pressure. Keep in mind what the response is! After you have treated the horse with PPS, we will try a fresh assessment and measure your effectiveness accordingly!

In the event that you provoke no response from your horse, and the back actually feels soft – perfect! I would like to congratulate you, because it is highly improbable that your horse is under any physical stress.

When you get no reaction from a back that feels really hard, you should seriously consider getting your horse to an experienced therapist.

You can contribute to the general feeling of well-being of an exceedingly strained horse by using PPS, but for complete healing, you will need some professional assistance.

21: Run your fingers alongside the spine to the front to test for tension in the elastic band.

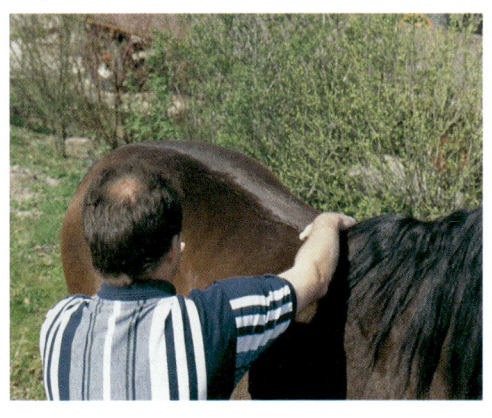

22: This horse reacts positively on the first test. The horse is not "ticklish", but has tension all over its body.

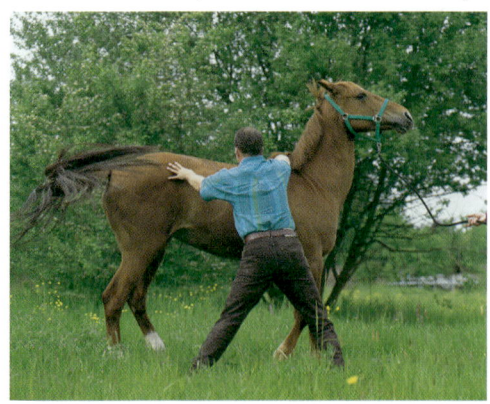

4.2. THE EIGHT REGIONS OF THE PRESSURE POINT SYSTEM

The following detailed descriptions of the pressure points and their locations will proceed from the front to the back. Whenever you are unsure how firmly you should "pole around" your horse with your fingertips (thumbs and fists are best employed), think of the experiment you did in Figures 5 and 6, and analyse again how hard you should press by using your forearm.

Acquaint yourself for the time being with the eight regions, and become motivated by your effectiveness in treating your horse frequently with PPS, but foremost get some proficient background to the regions.

Be careful that your fingernails are not too long – even if this is traumatic for the ladies, you should cut them short. Your fingertips must, after all, be able to detect problem zones under the skin of your horse, and eradicate them!

The intensive compression with your fingers may be quite demanding and unfamiliar. As with your horse, you too must gradually get used to PPS, but problems shared are problems halved. Rest assured, after the first correctly executed, fully comprehensive treatment of your horse, you will have some muscle aches of your own in your fingers and your arms.

Please remain faithful to our motto: "beat the cramps" by taking it slow, having frequent breaks, shaking your hands out and increasing your staying power carefully and little by little.

The duration of the first treatment should be approximately 40–50 minutes. Later on, you can rapidly inspect everything and need only treat the necessary problem areas. After treatment, the horse should be lightly exercised, so that the continued elevated blood flow can help with the removal of the oedema that has been massaged and needs to be cleared away.

4.2.1. REGION 1

LOCATION:
The topmost vertebra of the neck vertebrae (the atlas vertebra) is commonly recognised by the elevation just behind the poll (Figure 23) and therefore is a useful pointer.

This first point of treatment assists in the psychological relaxation of the horse by letting it take its head down, in that way peacefully receiving the treatment of the whole body.

Physical relaxation: the pressure point system

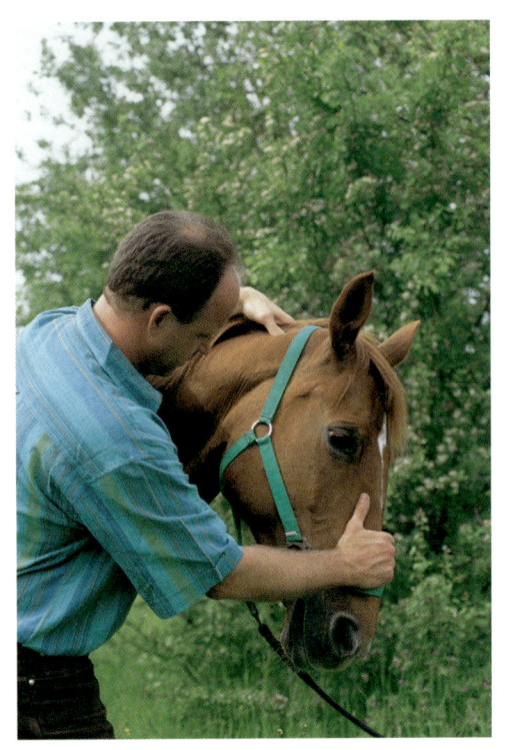

23: The first point must let the horse relax. This happens at best when the horse lowers his head. This first point is behind the atlas, at a 45-degree angle to the back. Push hard with the thumbs.

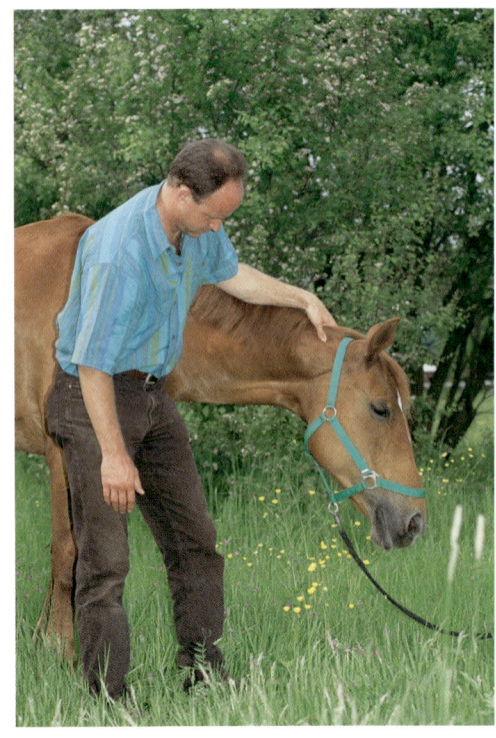

24: The horse has lowered his head and is obviously relaxed. Not every horse does this right at first; with patience and practice comes success.

You cannot force the horse's head down with muscle power: he must "let go" by himself. With this forward and down lengthening, the back muscles will relax, and even the vertebrae will become unconstrained. This point is just behind the bone of the atlas: starting from the poll, when you move your finger down along the mane, you will find, at an angle of about 45 degrees to the bone of the atlas, the attachment for two muscles.

Point 1 lies exactly in between these two muscles.

COMMENT:
Use the circling motion (anticlockwise) of your fingers that you have been applying since our first practical session. Wait patiently until the horse lets its head go really low; that makes everything increasingly easy.

Remember not to work for more than five minutes in one region. At first, you are only aiming for 1 per cent success! When your horse predominantly shakes his head in reaction to the pressure, you will know that you have found the exact

Physical relaxation: the pressure point system

point. Continue pressing firmly! Usually it will take some time for the horse to understand that it can and should relax (even for people relaxing is not generally that effortless …). One reliable indication that the horse is feeling happy and enjoying PPS is chewing. A good many horses will lower their heads straight away, while others will need much longer, maybe even more than one session – you have to be patient. The more you execute this manoeuvre with your horse, the sooner it will respond.

> With this you have arrived at a key position in the "centre of relaxation" for the horse – the secret of numerous "horse whisperers". This point can generally be employed in assorted circumstances when you need to release tension, for example, when having problems loading into a trailer.

Once you have stimulated the region at point 1, your endeavours will be supported by the release of the body's own stimulants. They will increase the flow of blood to the area for four or five hours, thus rendering the muscles and tendons more mobile, and transporting nutrients to the tissue and waste products away from it.

If your horse is relaxed, but his head is not completely lowered, there is no reason to be worried.

It is frequently the case that tension in other regions must be cleared away first (for example, in regions 2, 3 or 4, or at the elastic band). After three or four treatments you will find that the head will relax entirely and go down without any discomfort.

Remember the spider's web: all the muscles support and influence each other.

SAFETY:

This point should relax both the head and neck. Quietly hold the horse by its head collar. If the horse's head is held excessively high at first, do not try to reach the spot by standing on a stool or crate.

Try and use what little pressure you can exert from the ground. Remember, in one powerful movement you might be swept off your feet (and stool!).

Under no circumstances should you lean over the neck when it is lowered. Should your horse decide abruptly to lift his head, it normally happens extremely speedily and you will undoubtedly receive a blow to the chin, which you will not rapidly forget (after that you will never again lean over the neck when it is lowered …).

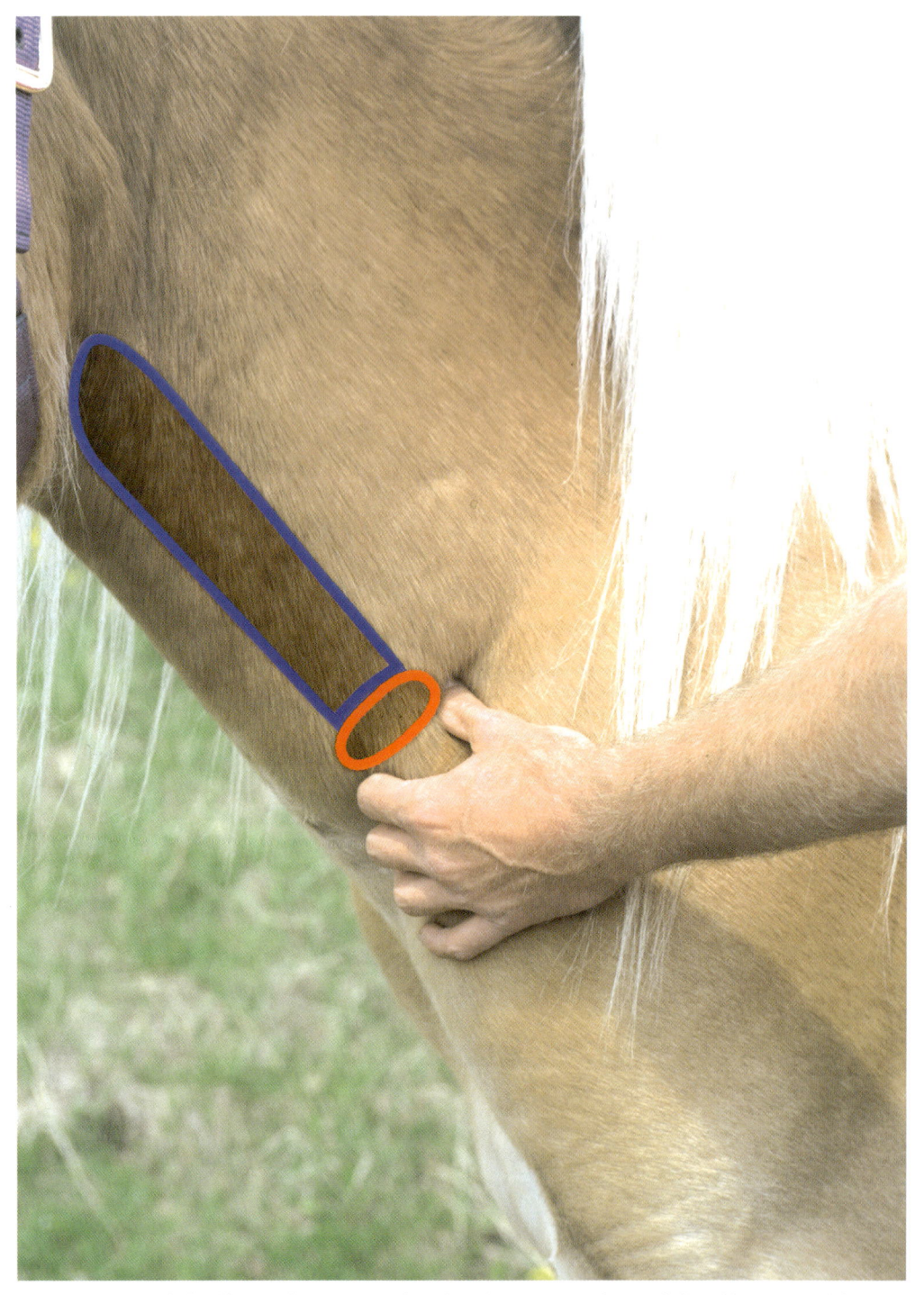

Physical relaxation: the pressure point system

25: The muscle marked in blue mainly causes trouble in the red area. Loosen the muscle by rubbing it up and down with your fist and then work in the red area using the circulating fingertip method.

38

4.2.2. REGION 2

In this region of the neck and shoulder we are interested in two locations, a and b.

LOCATION 2A:
In Figure 25 the blue lines mark a long muscle. Before you start applying PPS on this muscle, firmly rub the area four or five times, in the direction of the arrow, with your fist. You only physically work with your fingertips in the red designated area.

At the boundary of the muscle you will feel fibrous cords. Apply pressure to each of these cords, using the circular technique. Do not work for more than five minutes.

COMMENT:
Using your fist, you automatically awaken new key positions in the blue region. When you work in the red area, pay attention to your fingertips, explore the minute difference between tight and soft. Should you find you can detect the contrast before your five minutes has run out, you should discontinue.

If the pressure from your fingers varies individually and also in the different zones, you should not be too concerned that you are squeezing too hard or too soft. Apply as much pressure as it takes to be able to feel what is under the skin – after all, you want to experience the contrast between tight and soft. You should invariably compare the first sensation in your fingertips with the one you have after working on the muscles for a couple of minutes. By following these fundamental rules, you will rapidly develop a sensation as to the amount of compression you need to administer. Practice makes perfect, so carry on practising! With increasing experience you will be able to assess these circumstances effortlessly.

LOCATION 2B:
Region 2b lies inside the shoulder and you will find it at the junction of the neck and shoulder. Apply your fingertips in exactly the same way as in Figures 26 and 27. There are two great neck muscles that act on the shoulder joint through tendons. You must aim for these two tendinous insertions, because it is here that you must eliminate any possible oedema that has formed. In order to do that, it is important to insert your hand in the shoulder in the direction of the tendinous insertion.

COMMENT:
During the first few phases of this action, your hand will get tired. Most of the students on my workshops cannot persevere

Physical relaxation: the pressure point system

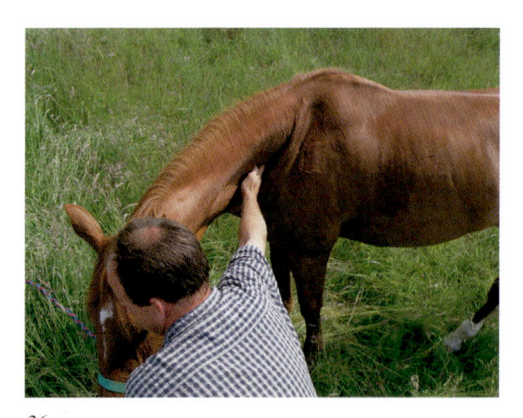

26

26/27/28: This looks impossible, but is really simple! Where the neck goes into the shoulder, just about in the middle, there is a door that will let you in. Try it! Pull the horse's head towards you and push the fingers on the shoulder. You will be surprised how easy it is to slip inside!
Massage the tendon attachments.
Your whole hand can disappear into the shoulder!

with PPS the first time, so severe are the aches in their fingers and muscles after only a few minutes. Shake them out energetically – let's continue!

You will have the equivalent sensation to that of a child that is trying to touch his toes with straightened legs for the first time. It will take some time, and beyond doubt several treatments before you actually reach your target. Put your right hand flat on the neck, so that the bottom part of it touches the shoulder blade. Now push the hand down and try carefully to disappear into the shoulder.

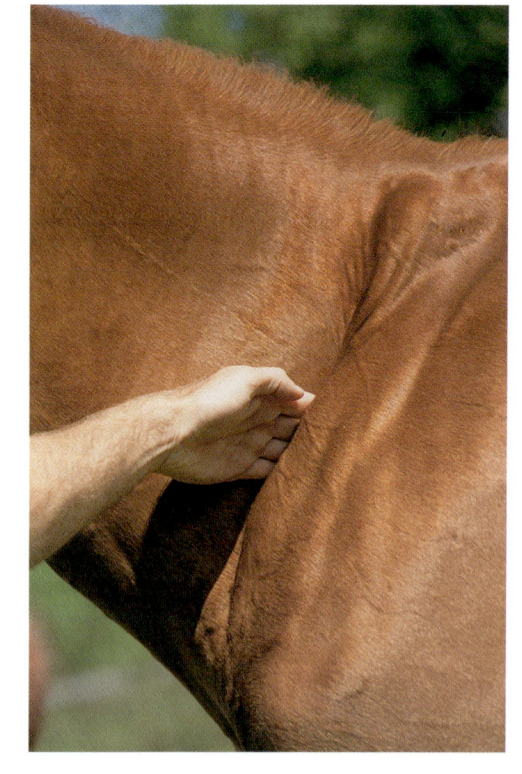

27

28

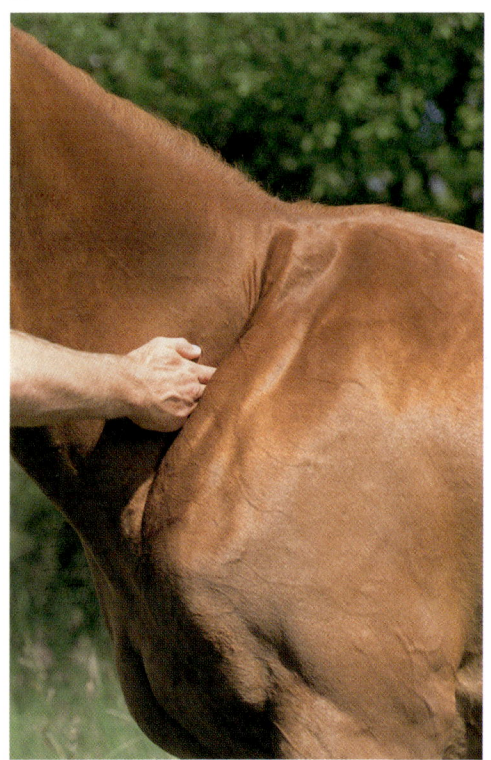

Physical relaxation: the pressure point system

By now you will be certain that you have arrived at a locked door. However, when you apply constant pressure and remain unrestricted yourself, you will find the doors opening gradually. Simply keep applying more pressure against the resistance. The horse will become increasingly loose and will give way with its head. Wait for that to happen before you attempt to go any deeper. Keep your eyes on the horse, notice its body language and respond accordingly.

It could take up to a few weeks before the door opens wide enough for your hand to disappear completely into the shoulder. You can then touch some single cords here and by applying pressure in a circular movement, loosen them up.

It is extremely helpful to pull the horse's head towards you, parallel to the shoulder, when you endeavour to penetrate the shoulder in this way.

SAFETY:

Over the years I have had occasional surprises while working in region 2b, so be on your guard! Try and build a kind of bony bridge between the horse and yourself, by supporting your hand on the horse's head and keeping your elbow fixed into your body. When the horse's head swings unannounced in your direction, it will be called to halt by your arm and not your face (in an unfortunate predicament, this could be a left hook to the chin…).

It can also happen that the horse is standing quite sensibly with lowered head, then something unexpected draws its attention and the horse stretches its head in the air. For such cases you should always hold the end of a lead rein in your hand, so that you– fingers in the head collar – do not get launched yourself, but can just let go of the head collar and still control the horse. As soon as the horse has learnt how pleasant PPS is, it will relax outright, appreciate the treatment and not be prone to any distractions.

29: Hold the horse by the head collar for your own safety. A sudden hook to the chin can be rather unpleasant…

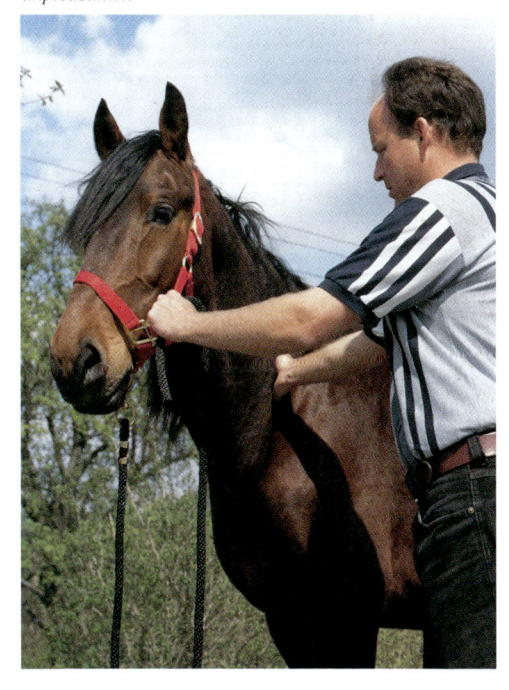

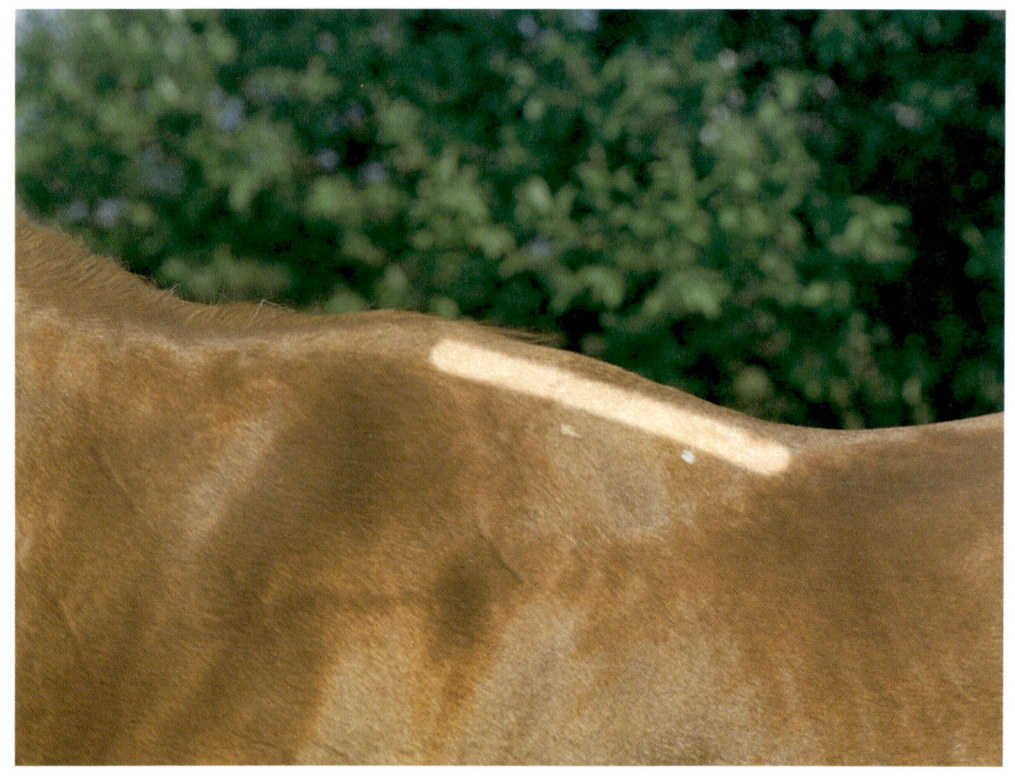

Physical relaxation: the pressure point system

30: The most important points of region 3 (withers) lie next to each other in the marked area.

4.2.3. REGION 3

LOCATION:
This region on the withers has a central importance to the pressure point system. This is where the body of the horse comes into contact with the rigid construction of the tree of the saddle while moving in three dimensions (front to back, up and down, left and right). The saddle and rider disposes acute pressure on the tendonous attachments, and not only when landing after a jump! In the lengthening of these tendons we find muscles that in turn become tendons that reach down into the lower forearm. Tightness in the withers can indirectly cause limitation in the movement of the lower forearm. (Tension that gives rise to shortening of muscles in the upper attachment, see chapter 3.3).

You can properly operate with your thumbs in this region. The light-coloured striation (Figure 30) lies just under the top of the vertebrae.

Physical relaxation: the pressure point system

COMMENT:

Get hold of the withers with both hands, thumbs on the side that is to be treated. Grasp the bony crest, move up or down the withers on the light-coloured striation shown in Figure 30, using circular pressure with your thumbs. Twitching of the skin, butting with the head and swishing of the tail (Figure 31) that you might notice in the beginning will cease with progressive treatment (your accomplishment with PPS!).

Horses with high withers are straightforward to treat in region 3. Horses with extremely low withers can be treated by placing one hand on top of the other and using the fingertips instead of the thumbs.

SAFETY:

Pay attention to your feet; with a big horse you have to stand really close and stretch your arms way up to grasp the withers if your horse has any tightness in this region (which in all likelihood is the case). He will not restrict himself to twitching his skin, but might trample around agitatedly, mind your feet! Head butts do not always have to be to the front and up (Figure 31) but nipping to the back is also possible.

A lot of horses suffer with complications in this area (for example saddle pressure) so you should beware of painful responses!

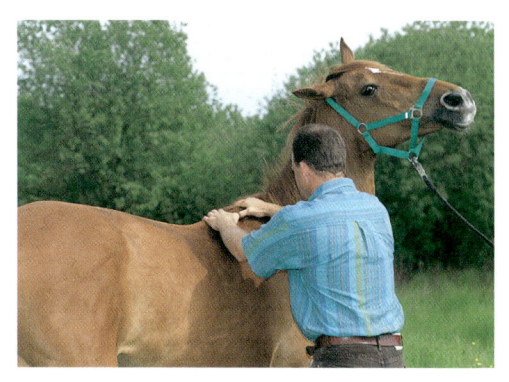

31: A badly fitting saddle is only one reason for problems in this area. Do not be surprised by reactions like head swinging, tail swishing etc. This area in particular will respond rapidly and the horse will calm down quickly.

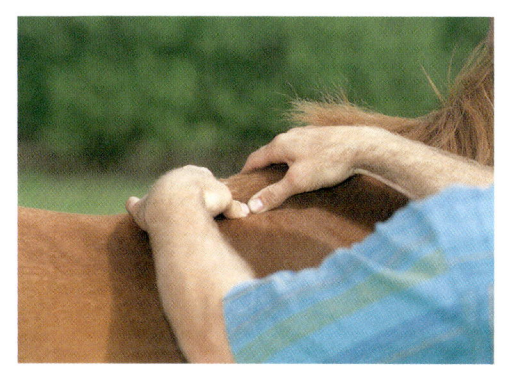

32: The attachments of the tendons in this area are very close together and can be easily massaged by holding the bony part with your fingers while moving in circles with the thumbs.

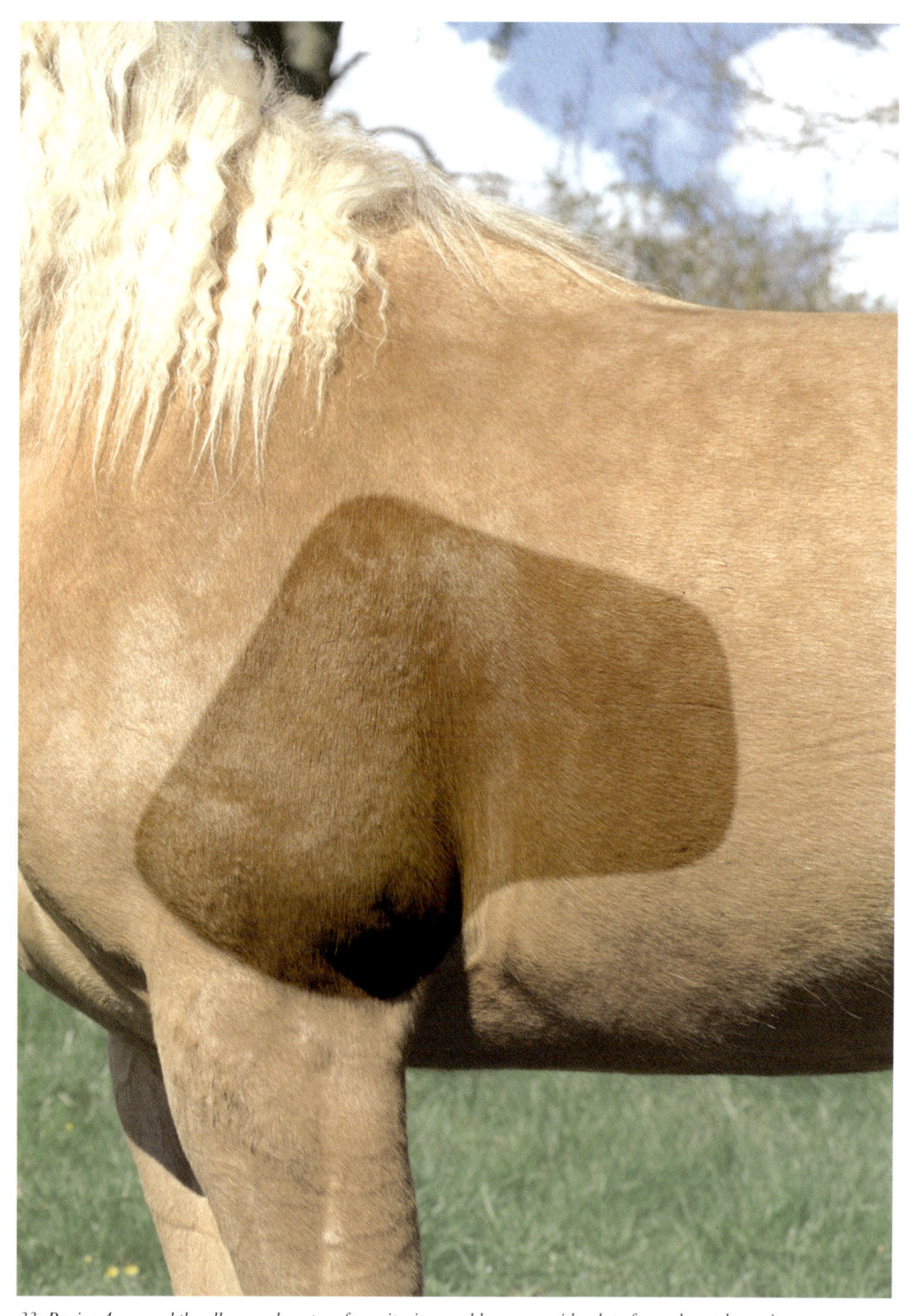

Physical relaxation: the pressure point system

33: Region 4, around the elbow and centre of gravity, is a problem area with a lot of muscle-tendon units.

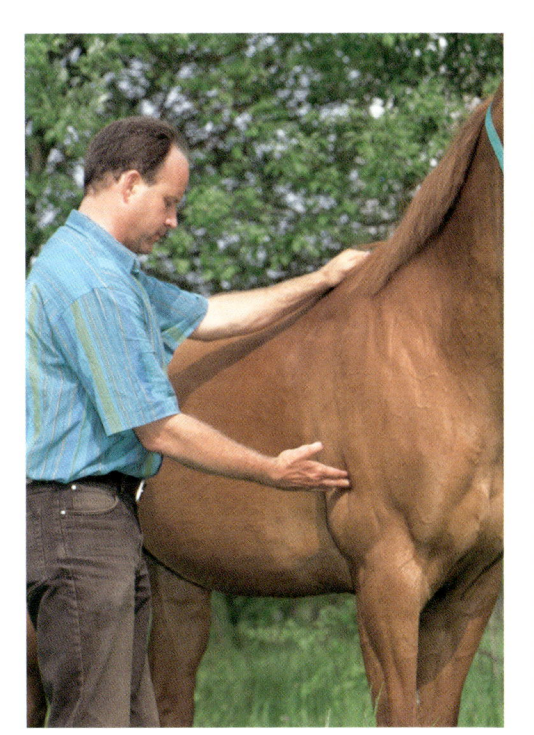

Physical relaxation: the pressure point system

34: Poke with straightened fingers the whole area of region 4, while observing the reaction of the horse.

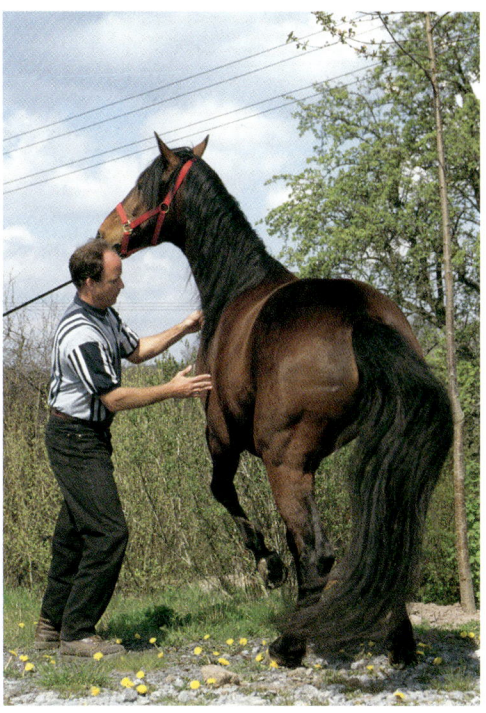

35: The horse's reaction depends on the degree of tension, from tail swishing to rearing: the horse is not just "ticklish". You will notice the difference in behaviour after one treatment.

4.2.4. REGION 4

LOCATION:

The area of the elbow and the centre of gravity for the horse is where a formidable collection of muscles and tendons meet. This region (Figure 33) is a particularly susceptible stress area in a lot of horses and painful stiffness frequently makes an appearance, even when grooming your horse.

Exactly as you have experimented at the beginning of this book, in this region you must look for the nerve ending – the doorbell. You start at the top of the region and poke around step by step on the horse, to detect which bell rings the loudest.

Observe your horse carefully: where does he demonstrate the strongest reaction? (Figure 35). Commence your labour in this region and continue to the other regions.

It is indeed possible that the horse can be so acutely strained that it will exhibit an extreme reaction even to a soft touch (some will bellow, or squeak like a mare in season). Such a sad and miserable pre-

Physical relaxation: the pressure point system

> Your horse is not ticklish, he has tension! Treat your horse and you will have no more "ticklish" reactions – neither when grooming nor when saddling.

dicament makes it impossible for you to locate any oedema under the skin. The best you can do is to get the circulation going in this extensive area. Apply your fist (Figure 36) and rub energetically, using all your strength, or at least as arduously as the horse will allow, this way and that way across region 4, up and down, backwards and forwards. Support yourself with your elbow tucked in your body: that way you can use even more strength. This extensive treatment will loosen bogged down fibres and numerous small superficial muscles and tendons will be able to loosen up. Treat the entire area four or five times, until the blood flow has been elevated and then once again examine the whole of region 4.

What do you think? Is there a small improvement? Your horse will experience some relief.

You can either repeat the whole procedure or inspect the area, using your fingertips, for more concrete signs of oedema that is fixed in between the tissue. You will recognise them as small, honeycomb-textured lumps, up to the size of a fingernail. Clear them away by employing circular pressure.

COMMENT:

If region 4 is still tight after the above treatment has been executed (this is possible when it is an old problem), simply persevere with the manipulation. Sooner or later, you will be successful, finding the ringing bell and its exact location and being able to eliminate it entirely.

Within the framework of my workshops, I can demonstrate the longer and shorter sections of the muscles in this area, but I have to emphasise that effective treatment does not centre on the anatomic details, but on the actual treatment in the horse and the fundamental effort put into the short (Figure 37, red) and long (blue) muscles in this region.

36: If there is a severe reaction to treatment in region 4, it is advisable to use your fist at first.

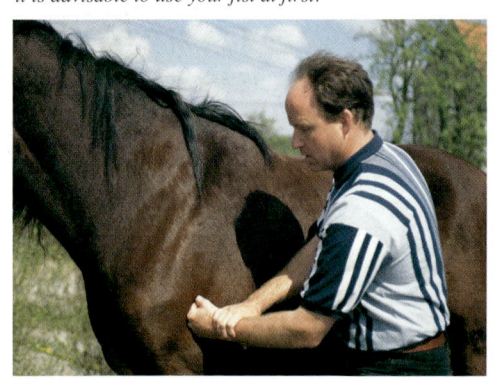

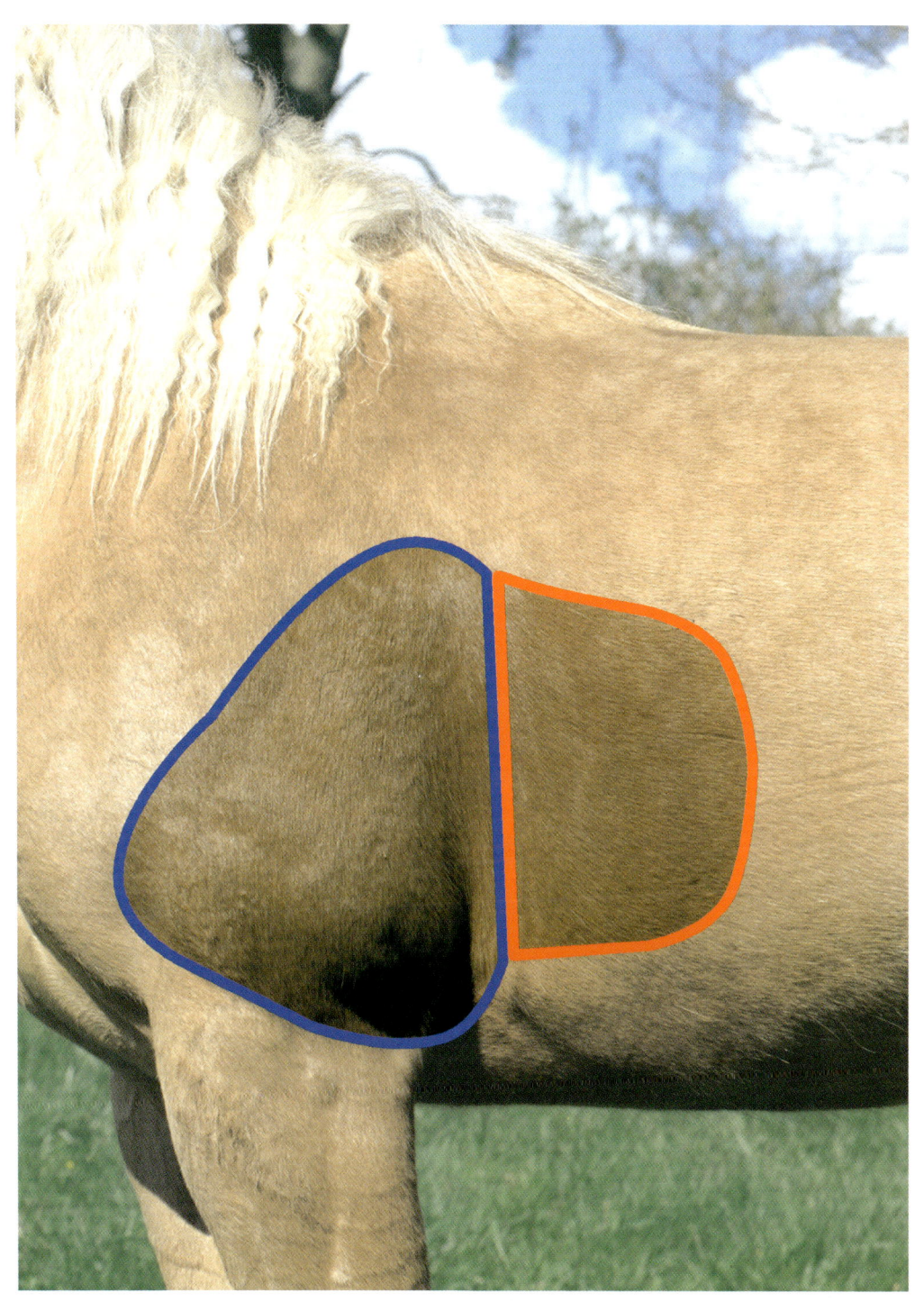

Physical relaxation: the pressure point system

37: Region 4: In order to find the longer muscles in the blue area, use the technique described in Figure 13. The smaller muscles in the red area can be treated using both the fingers and the fist, Fig. 8.

Physical relaxation: the pressure point system

Short (red): When you work in the red space, simply replace your fingertips with your fist! This way you will capture and eliminate a vast number of small problems. Later on you can interchange this technique with your fingertips again and extinguish the last sporadic reprisals that got left behind.

Long (blue): There is not in actual fact an abundant amount of long muscles in this area, but it is worthwhile to look for the doorbell over here as well. Press down with your fingertips on the surface where your horse displayed the most compelling behaviour.

Identify the body of the muscle and, still pressing down, move your fingers left and right and then down, until you feel the end of the muscle body.

STOP! Start administering PPS in the usual, circular manner (for not longer than five minutes) on the tendon.

That may sound rather complicated, but the only thing that can go amiss is that you "do not hear" the doorbell (or misinterpret it as a skin twitch ...) and have to recommence your search.

SAFETY:
Severely strained horses will resort to extensive evasive manoeuvres, so keep an eye on that. When they are in acute pain you can also expect nipping and kicking (as they do when they have flies under their bellies).

Your horse is not ticklish, only under adverse tension. You can help your horse with PPS.

CROUP AND HINDQUARTERS

The formidable muscles of the "engine" in the horse's movement have immense demands made upon them.

Back problems (e.g. caused by a poorly fitting saddle) can extend into the gluteal muscles and affect the overall performance of the horse.

Corresponding to the magnitude of the bulk of muscle in this area, you will uncover a formidable quantity of pressure points, but experience has taught me that the treatment of fewer regions is sufficient to achieve results.

Physical relaxation: the pressure point system

For the activity surrounding the hindquarters it is essential to emphasise the importance of safety measures. They are valid for all points inside regions 5–8! It is better, at the onset, to be too careful, to leap away too early ten times, than once too late! You would after all like to give your horse the enjoyment of being massaged more than once ...

It is advisable, when you undertake to work on the hindquarters, to support yourself with a stretched-out arm on the body of the horse, while you use the other to treat the horse. This way you will be aware when the horse prepares to kick, by the way he tenses his muscles in his body, and can swiftly get out of harm's way. Besides, this way the horse can catapult the therapist away from the danger zone with its mere movement, before it can give you a "hit".

In this area, it is essential for you to keep an eye on your horse's body language! The body language is of prime importance to coherent treatment (annoyed reactions point to the tension areas; peaceful, positive feedback demonstrates the effectiveness of your treatment), and in the hindquarters you are exposed to above-average danger.

Never trust anyone who says: "my horse never kicks".

Horses will try to remove anything or anyone that causes pain to them, not necessarily in a malicious way, but purely out of reflex. Move away instantly, as soon as you suspect the horse might kick.

If it really does kick, leave it in peace for a moment, and then commence your activity again, this time with less pressure. After a few successful treatments the tension in your horse will start to diminish. Then you can employ solid pressure again, because the suffering will ease more and more with the application of PPS, and your horse will have no more reason to kick you.

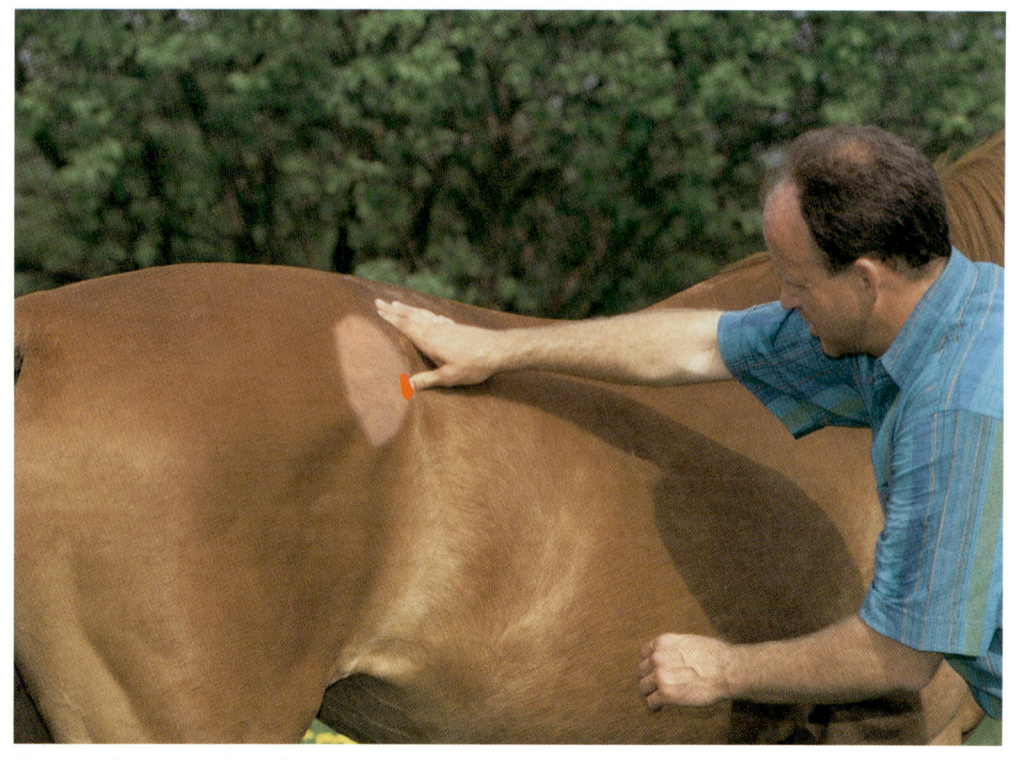

Physical relaxation: the pressure point system

38: Region 5 comprises three different areas. As a pointer we start at the hipbone. The red spot is location 5a, which lies between the last rib and the hipbone.

4.2.5. REGION 5

This region comprises three different areas that can vary according to the breed and constitution of your horse. To find the three areas, always use the red mark in Figure 38 as your pointer.

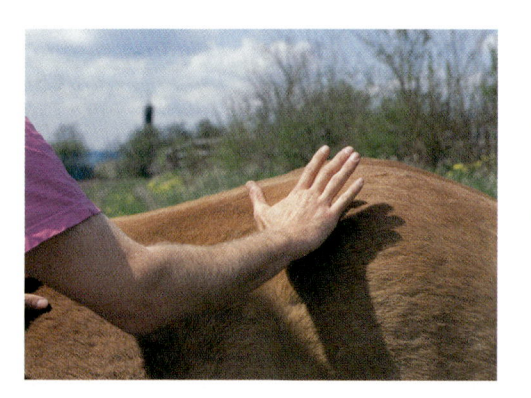

LOCATION 5A:
Horses particularly enjoy pressure on a point that you can identify between the last rib and the hipbone.

The best way to find it is to place your thumb on the hipbone, let it slide to the front of the horse and press from the bottom of the hipbone.

39: It is difficult to find the hipbone of the heavy breeds. Slap around the area and you will soon find the bone under soft tissue.

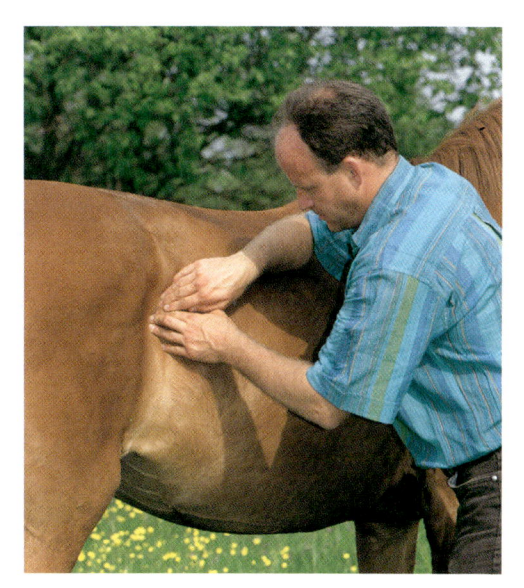

Physical relaxation: the pressure point system

40: The horse must have weight on all four legs when treating location 5b.

There you should find, according to the anatomy of the horse, a small tendon.

COMMENT:
With corpulent, extremely muscular or cold-blooded horses, you can have a difficult time finding even the hipbone.

When you slap the area energetically you might have a chance of finding a bony landmark (Figure 39).

LOCATION 5B:
This point lies close behind the ribs where you will find a flat ligament that can be massaged with the fingers.

COMMENT:
Ultimately, this point should be pushed with all your power, but make sure the horse stands with weight on all four feet.

LOCATION 5C:
Use the highlighted mark in Figure 42 to find this area. Work through the area using circular movements with all your fingers.

COMMENT:
In location 5c we are not attempting to find a single point, but want to stimulate the whole area.

41: To exert more pressure, you can strengthen the hand by putting the other one on top.

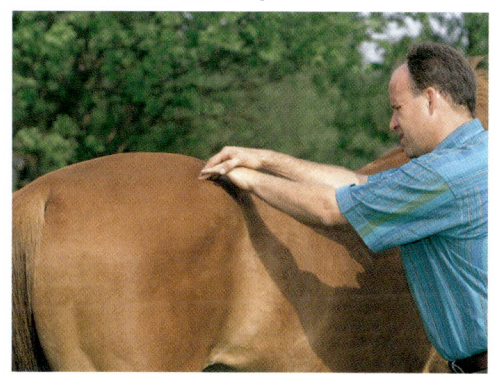

42: Use the fingertip technique to work in the area of location 5c. If you find a tight spot, simply massage a bit longer in this area.

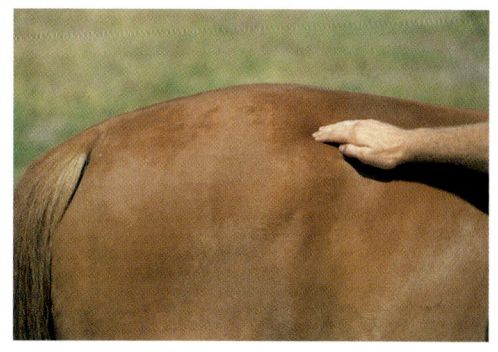

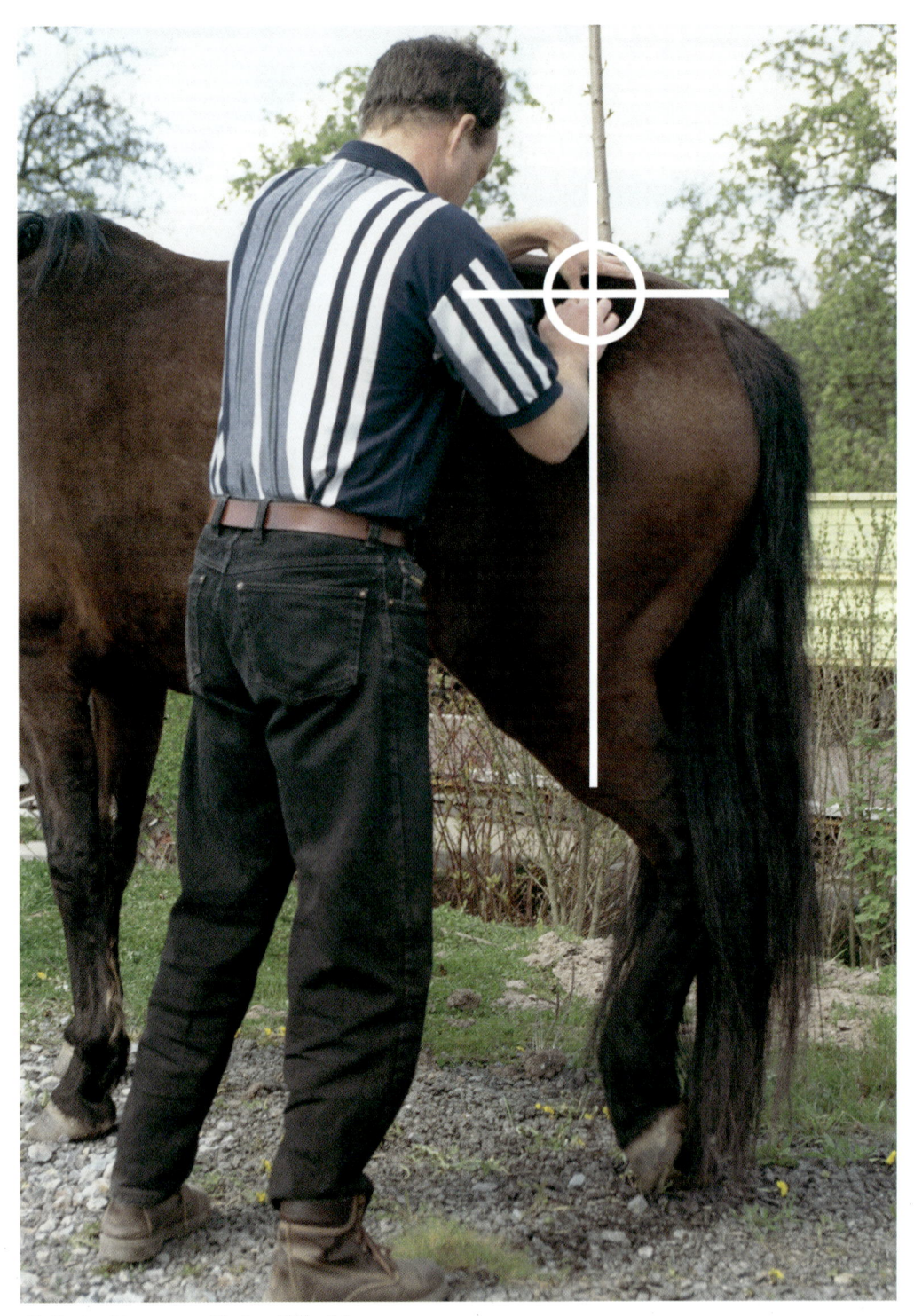

Physical relaxation: the pressure point system

43: Region 6 is on top and in the middle of the croup.

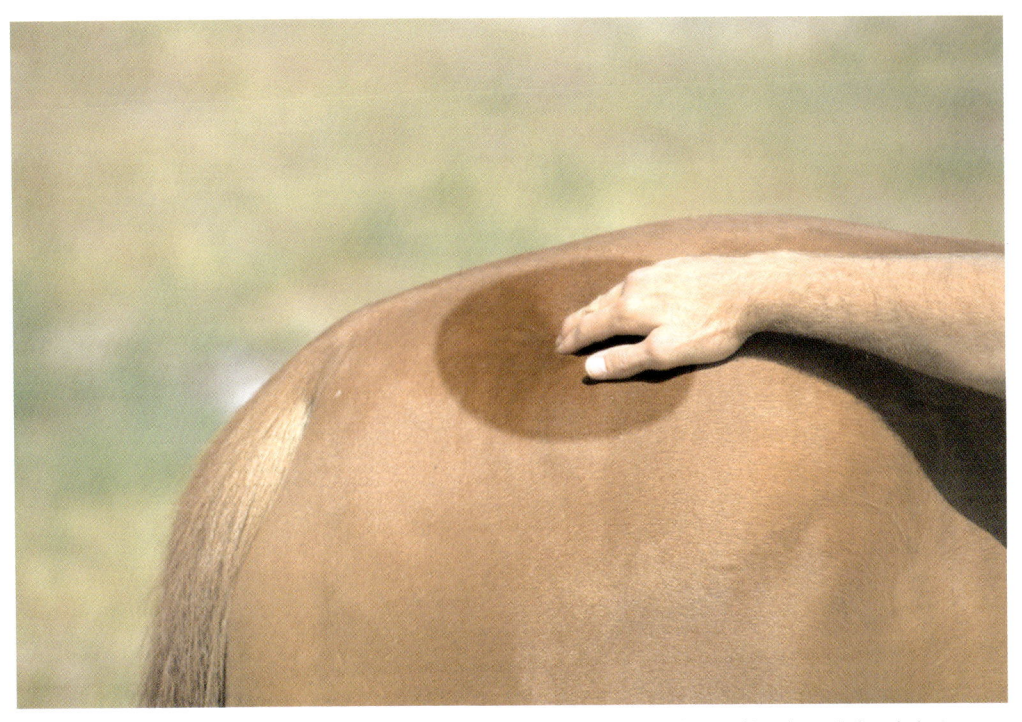

Physical relaxation: the pressure point system

44: This is where region 6 is. Once again it is not about finding a single point, but working through the whole area.

4.2.6. REGION 6

LOCATION
The line in Figure 43 shows the middle of the hindquarters.

Starting at the highest point near the spine, work your way through region 6. Slightly to the back you will come across a border between two muscles. This is the middle of region 6 (Figure 44)

COMMENT:
If your horse reacts severely at this point, it is advisable to get the opinion of a PPS expert. When you slide your hand over the rounding of the croup, you will most likely not notice anything. The area is round and smooth. After 10–15 cm, using slightly bent fingers, you will find it deepening; this is exactly the spot where you should press.

Once more this is not a single point, but the whole of this lower area.

Later on, using the other hand on top can strengthen the pressure but only once you are sure that the horse has relaxed completely! (The horse takes its weight off the leg and lowers its head.)

In a short while you will be able to find this point in your sleep!

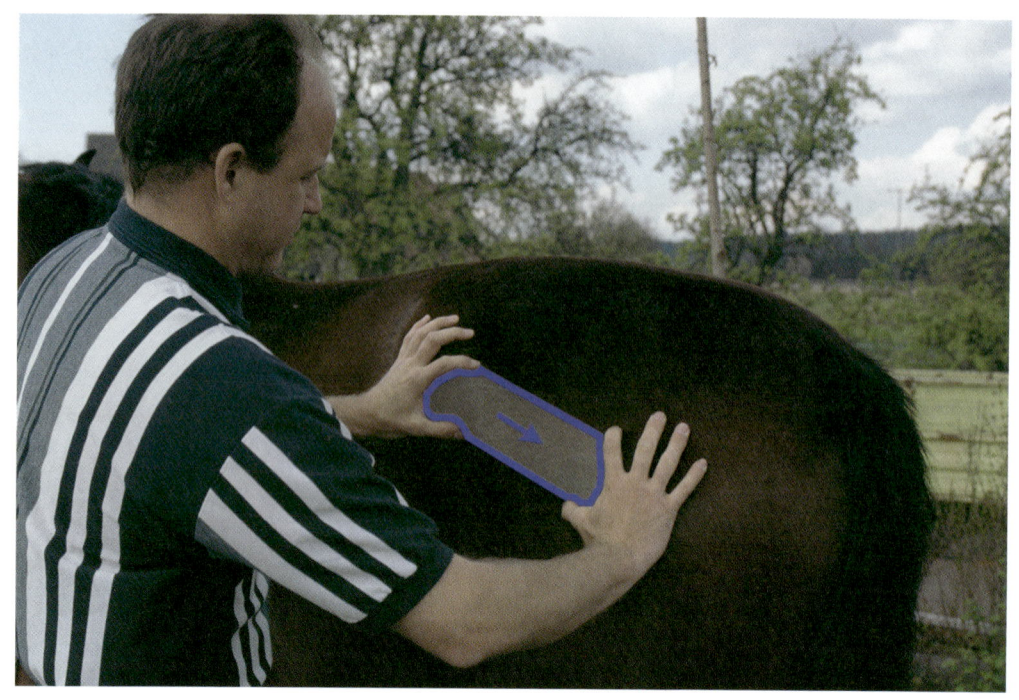

Physical relaxation: the pressure point system

45: This is region 7. You work in this area (as in region 2a) with your fist.

46: Use circular movement with the fingertips along the blue line.

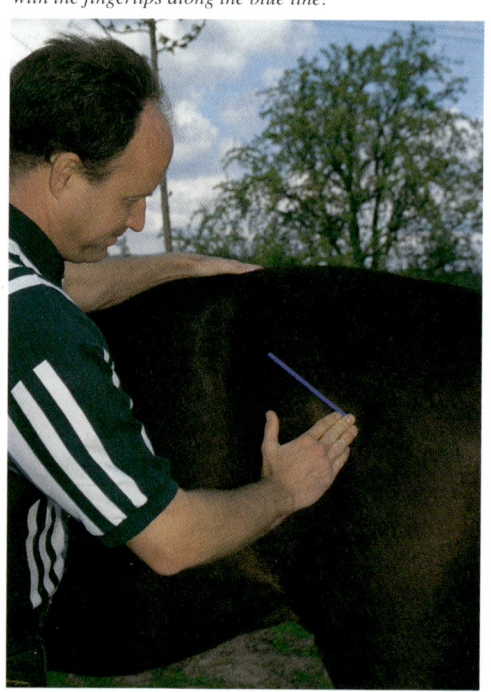

4.2.7. REGION 7

LOCATION

In Figure 45 you can see exactly where the muscle is. Massage with your fist along this area in the direction of the arrow. Follow the blue line in Figure 46 using circular movements with the fingertips.

COMMENT:

Pay attention to what you are feeling. When you work inside the blue area and find something hard, linger on that for a while before moving on to the rest. If you start too far back, you can feel a bone; only work in front of this bone!

Physical relaxation: the pressure point system

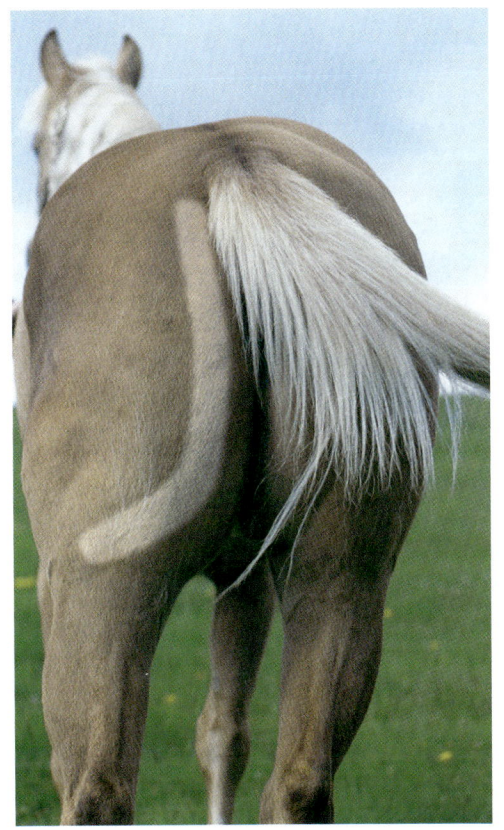

47. This area on the hindquarters has many pressure points; all are to be massaged with the fingertips using the circular technique.

4.2.8. REGION 8

Great care must be taken with your safety, as you will be working mainly behind the horse in region 8.

There is more than one pressure point in the area of the seat bone. You must use the fingertips in a circular movement when working on this area. A very tense horse will tip his pelvis when you start working on him.

The easiest point to find is 8b and the rest are simple to identify from there.

8b) Press around the area of the seat bone. It is easy to find and only light pressure should be used to work in this area.

8a) Approximately 1–2 cm above 8b you will find 8a. When you press on this point you will feel a flattening of tissue,

48. You start the work in region 8 with point 8b; this point is easy to find with the help of the seat bone! This bone is directly under your finger, so the pressure should not be as firm as with the other points in region 8.

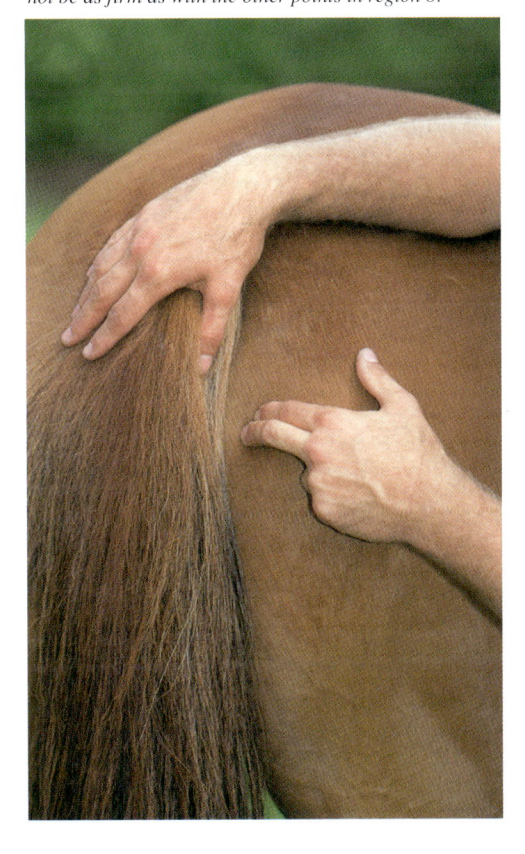

Physical relaxation: the pressure point system

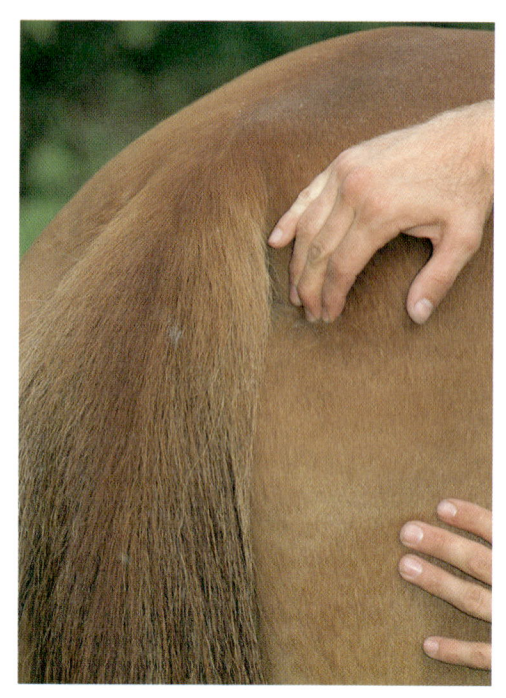

49. Point 8b lies a few centimetres above 8a.

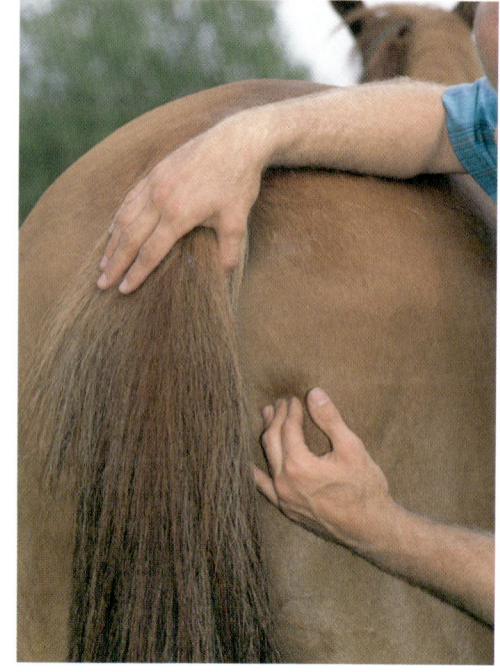

50. Some centimetres below the seat bone you will find 8c.

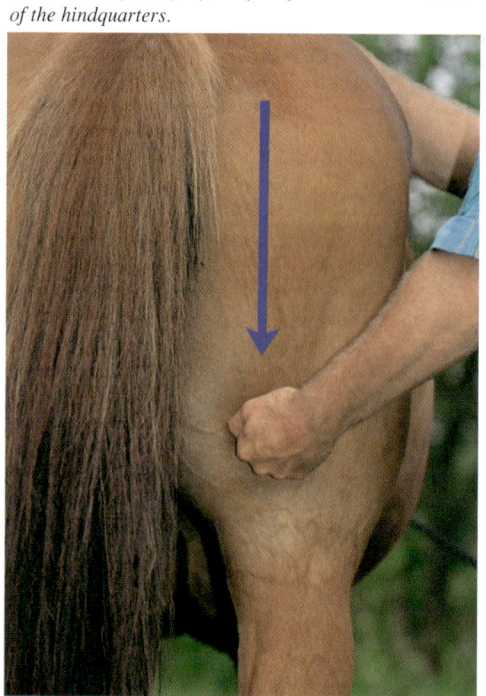

51. Point 8d: powerfully rub your fist down the muscles of the hindquarters.

52. Here, at the end of the hindquarters, you will find point 8e.

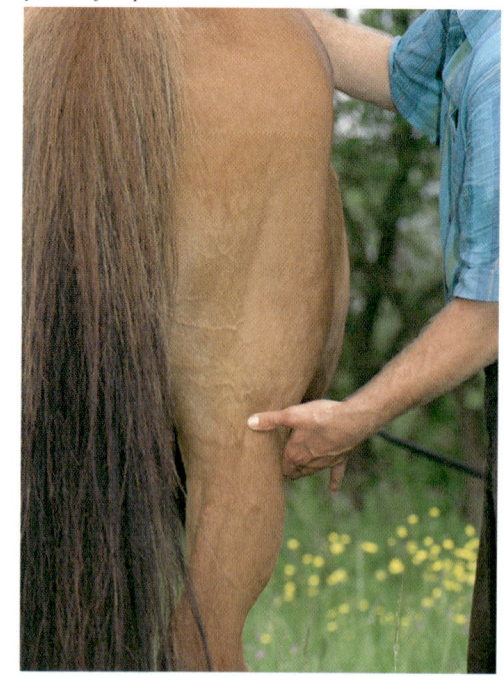

where you can work with normal pressure again.

8c) From point 8b, move your fingers 4–5 cm lower; this area always feels very soft, but in a small circle you can feel a few hard tendons. This is where you must work, but remember, no more than five minutes!

8d) Horses that are fit and well muscled make it easy for you to find this area. When the horse is not in such good condition, simply rub over the shown area (Figure 51) and try to find the muscle in this way.

8e) Simply follow the blue line shown in Figure 51; at the end of this line is point 8e (Figure 52). Massage the area carefully with the thumbs, using a circular movement.

4.3. THE CONCLUDING TEST

Naturally you have to treat both sides of your horse with the pressure point system, but it is interesting to compare the two sides with each other after treating only one side; test the "ticklish" areas of your horse. After just one treatment the difference – even if it is only small – is already noticeable.

Several intensive treatments are needed if the horse has severe tightness. Once your horse is comfortable or completely loosened up, you only need to do regular checks on the eight regions to keep stubborn tensions at bay.

> After treatment of both sides it is important to exercise your horse for 15–20 minutes within the first three hours. This way the circulation can get rid of the residue that came out of the muscles and their fibres.

Physical relaxation: the pressure point system

4.4. WHEN AND HOW OFTEN SHOULD YOU USE PPS?

You now know how to find tension in your horse using the "doorbell" technique. A good time for a check is just before you go riding, or any time you have the impression that your horse has some slight problem under saddle or in hand.

Always remember to warm up and move the previously strained and partly inactive muscles in order for them to work with their colleagues.

It requires at least one to two months of basic work for the treated horse to regain his balance.

During this time it is recommended to use PPS to keep the blood flow at a high level, and the muscles loose, in order for the healing process to proceed without any extra pressure.

Test the eight regions once or twice a week for any tension. With a little practice it is possible to find other areas of tension in the horse; you can treat them like any other area.

Remember that 1 per cent success is a big achievement!

You will in all probability be so encouraged by your accomplishments that you will wander beyond the eight regions, detect reactions and be able to eliminate them. Do not fear, you cannot hurt the horse with only your fingertips!

4.5. EXTENDED REFERENCE TO THE INDIVIDUAL REGIONS

I did not want to overload you with too much information on the single regions at the beginning, but now that you have some practical experience, I would like to add some information. This extra knowledge will help to deal with further problems that I often have to cope with as well in my work.

Once you are sure of the regions and their locations, this chapter can deepen your knowledge. When you encounter any difficulty in one or another region, do not give in; simply continue as best you can. Bearing in mind that all muscles are connected (the spider's web!) you will find it easier to achieve something as you go along.

My students all confirm that they are capable of loosening tension in all eight regions after as little as five or six treatments, whatever their previous experience in this field.

Physical relaxation: the pressure point system

4.5.1. REGION 1

Many people have problems finding the first point; this is not unusual, seeing that you have not done anything of this nature before and that the first point is the most difficult one of them all to find.

Maybe you are not sure whether you have found the exact spot, are not sure how hard to press, or are worried that you might hurt the horse.

If you cannot find this point, do not be concerned, simply work as well as you can and with the experience you get in the other regions, you will know exactly how to tackle the horse. The horses will also start to value the treatment and will be more accommodating, especially at point one.

Over the years I have often found that horses have more problems in this area than anywhere else. This can be from a fall as a foal or play as a yearling, or a bang on the head in the box or stable. Be aware that you can get some hefty reactions in this area.

If the situation does not get any better after four or five intensive treatments with PPS and stretching (chapter 5.4), it might be sensible to have the area examined by a vet.

4.5.2. REGION 2

2a) Does your horse flinch when you press in this area? Rub the area with your fist to raise the blood flow in the tissue. If the horse has real problems in the neck and shoulder area, none of the work done at the attachment of the tendon will be of any use unless you have loosened the neck muscles to some degree.

Use your fist on a regular basis, even when your horse has reacted well to the therapy.

The muscles will be positively stimulated and within four or five treatments you will notice that the muscles are softer and also stay supple.

> Be careful: When using firm pressure, which the horse may need, you can actually rub off sections of your own skin without noticing!

2b) If the horse continues to react strongly in this area, this most probably means that there is still tightness in area 4 or 5. Think of the spider's web and simply try and loosen up the rest of the body as best you can.

The most difficult part in this area is to push your hand into this outwardly closed region! Whether you do it with the back of your hand or fingers first, just try it and use the way you are more at ease with.

Do not use any force! Simply push and then wait for the horse to let you in. When the head lowers, it is normally a sign that all is well, push a little more and move in deeper. How deep? Theoretically you can push your whole hand into the shoulder; watch your horse carefully, when he lowers his head and turns towards you it is a good sign that you have reached the spot. You can also lightly pull the head forwards sideways; the horse relaxes more with this little aid.

4.5.3. REGION 3

One of the most important points of PPS will help you to test a horse when you are out to buy. Tension in this area automatically leads to problems elsewhere and is almost always founded in pressure from the saddle.

"My saddle fits" or "I use a thick pad" is something I hear often, but the reaction of the horse shows the opposite. Do remember: small tensions in the tendons often stay hidden and reactions only become obvious when about 30 per cent damage has been done. Rider and saddle put enormous pressure on the withers.

When you find bigger complications in this region it could well be from previous owners and saddles, but if these problems do not get better with PPS, you should seriously consider a new saddle.

Since that tension has physiological causes, a gel pad will not solve the problem of saddle pressure: the concentrated pressure on a small surface will push the gel to one side and although you have done it with the best of intentions, the saddle will continue pinching! Several resourceful entrepreneurs offer computerised examinations to solve the problem of a badly-fitting saddle; using PPS may take longer, but it is free!

Examine region 3 with all the power you have in your finger! You will soon see if any tension is present, for the horse will twitch the skin in the area as if to rid himself of a fly.

If you encounter strong reaction in this area, it is best not to ride the horse for two or three weeks. After complete easing of the tautness you can test the saddle for any difficulties.

4.5.4. REGION 4

Initially it is difficult to know which of the many muscles in this area is the one with the problem. It is therefore important to test the whole area around the elbow and centre of gravity, and especially where the girth lies. If any unease is present it will show itself with twitching of the skin.

When the horse has problems during grooming, or shows any reaction when you check the area, it means that there is tension that causes pain! It may seem inconceivable that a big horse should show discomfort from the touch of a brush, but that is unfortunately the case when a horse has had tension in this region for many years.

Eventually the pain becomes so severe that the horse lashes out with teeth and feet at even a soft touch of the hand or brush. Do you know a horse that does this? Examine him in region 4; the cause of this behaviour often lies in the tension there and you literally have the remedy in your hands. Unfortunately, no prediction can be made as to the exact length of time needed to eliminate the strained areas. Simply treat the horse every second day with PPS, make notes of the reactions you get and derive pleasure from the little improvements you begin to notice.

If your horse happens to show the extreme behaviour discussed above, you should have a lot of patience and take your time. Within four or five treatments the horse will already feel healthier and his muscles will relax more with each treatment.

In severe cases the horse will have aching muscles the next day; after all, the muscles have only been working at half of their capacity for years and now have the possibility to function properly again. If your horse has a slight lameness after treatment there is no reason for worry; move your horse lightly, massage some more, get the blood flow going and set the muscle in motion again. This will build up the muscle and the horse will be able to move again without any pain.

Bear in mind that the horse must show some improvement within six weeks of treatment. If this is not the case, you should get professional help to examine your horse for any further problems. Once your horse is fully loosened up, it will be no problem to keep him that way by using the eight-point PPS and stretching that will be explained later.

Physical relaxation: the pressure point system

4.5.5. REGION 5

5a) Seeing that this muscle-tendon unity is under more strain than any other region, it is not always easy to recognise a knot in this area; simply carry on working, you cannot do any harm.

Increased experience will teach you the difference between natural and unnatural tension. Try this particular area on eight to ten different horses; this will give you a better idea when you return to your own horse as to what it should feel like.

> AT THIS STAGE I HAVE TO REPEAT THE WARNING: Even with the most peaceful horses you have to remember that pain can make them react in an unexpected way. Support yourself against the horse with an outstretched arm and jump out of harm's way the moment you feel the horse tense up his muscles ...

5b) Many horses react indignantly when groomed in this area. Rub the area firmly with your fist and you will see an improvement of behaviour within a few treatments.

In order for you to find this area the horse must stand with weight equally distributed on all four legs. When the horse takes its weight off one hind leg (a sign of relaxation), you must push him back so that his weight is on all four legs, until you are sure that you can find this point even with a relaxed leg. The feeling of well-being achieved in this area often makes the horses grunt, especially when there is extensive tension. The animals are obviously relieved and express it; a beautiful confirmation of your work with PPS.

5c) Reactions in this area are common when tension spreads from the back. The vertebrae will lower slightly when you press on different points in this area; simply massage this area for one or two minutes, until you feel it going softer.

4.5.6. REGION 6

When your horse is well muscled or even fat, it will not be easy to find this point. For the best results, study Figure 43 and work in this general area. Within a few treatments the muscles of the hindquarters will be more relaxed and you will be able to find the point more easily.

4.5.7. REGION 7

Once you have some practice you can spot tension in this area with the naked eye; the muscle looks tight and isolated when the horse moves. By observing this area you will notice how this impression will disappear within a few treatments.

To loosen the tissue at first, rub the area firmly with your fist before doing detailed work with the fingertips. When this is not enough to loosen extremely tight tissue, you may punch the area lightly with the same amount of power you can stand on your own body. Once the tissue is loosened this extreme measure is no longer needed and the treatment can be started with PPS.

4.5.8. REGION 8

8a) Unfortunately this area always feels soft, even when strained. With successful manipulation this point might look somewhat deeper.

Remember our spider's web: all muscles are connected and even the smallest improvement in one muscle will help the others. Press this point for at least one minute, even when you do not feel any difference!

8b) The seat bone lies directly under this point, so it is not necessary to press as hard in this area.

Pay attention to hardened sections in this area; the tendons of region 8 are often under such tension that they feel like extremely tight shoelaces. Upon discovering such a shoelace, massage the area for one or two minutes until you feel it softening.

It is possible that you may not find anything at all, but some horses have severe tension in the hindquarters.

Stimulate the areas and take care that they are soft and the blood flow is activated. The problems will not disappear within a day, but will become diminished each time.

8c) Throughout the book I have been trying to explain the PPS as simply as possible and to describe what you should feel in the different regions. In almost all horses, region 8 should be elastic and pliable; when it is tight and somewhat thicker, this is a sure sign of tension.

8d) Horses with problems in this area will often react by tilting the pelvis. The muscle-tendon units will be hard as rock and your hand will be unable to make a dent in it. This will change within a few sessions of treatment.

Physical relaxation: the pressure point system

When this area is acutely strained you can start with light pushing of your fists, you might even need a few sessions for this. Your horse will soon feel relieved and less tempted to kick you because it hurts. BUT BE CAREFUL!

8e) This is another area where you can feel plenty of "shoelaces", and experience has taught that you can achieve success even in horses that are not as strained.

Right, you have pressed enough using your fingers! It is time to give your arms a rest!

> Problems in 8d/e are often a result of tension in regions 5c and 6. Concentrate on 5c and 6 and the problems in 8d/e will be less.

5. ADDITIONAL INFORMATION AND GYMNASTIC EXERCISES FOR YOUR HORSE

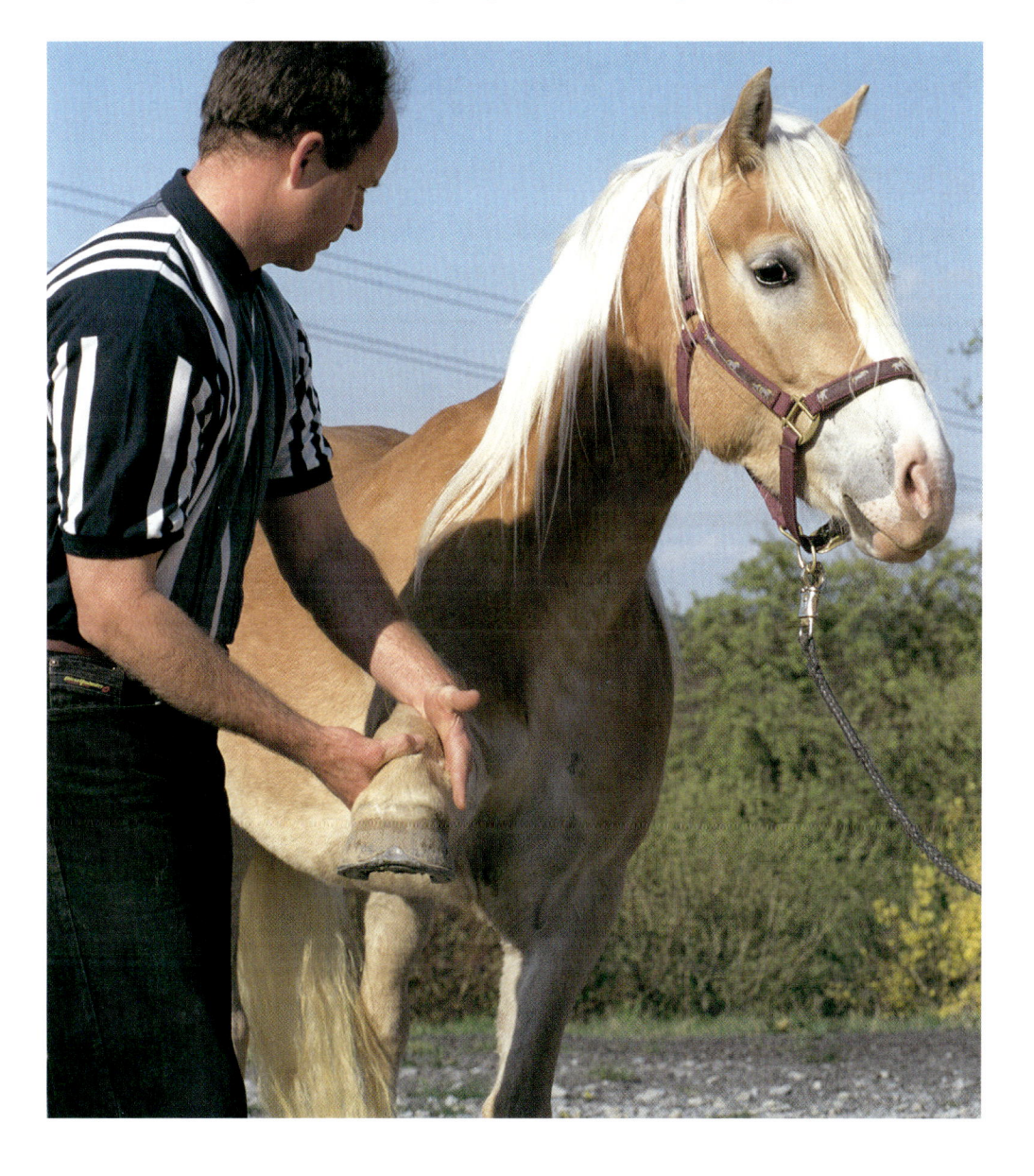

Additional information and gymnastic exercises

You can achieve a great deal with PPS when your horse has problems with tension. In this chapter I will suggest further possibilities to reduce the risk of strain. Some of these exercises, for example the stretching, can become part of your daily grooming.

Other exercises like the walk on a slope take more time, but are useful with specific problems. I would like to help you to observe as much as possible, for everything you do will influence your horse in a certain way and it is often small things that have big influences on the horse.

I once treated a horse that had been in a serious accident, and after two years of loving care we managed to get him in fine fettle again. His owner treats him with PPS, warms him up and cools him down and does everything possible for his health. That, however, did not stop the horse from going lame each time after being worked. Vets thought it was arthritis, rheumatism or delayed reaction to the accident. Everyone tried everything possible.

One morning I arrived at the stable early and discovered quite by accident that a well-meaning groom was giving the horse three times the normal amount of feed!

Once this was rectified the horse was better within days. So, do pay attention to small, seemingly harmless details when you have a problem.

Additional information and gymnastic exercises

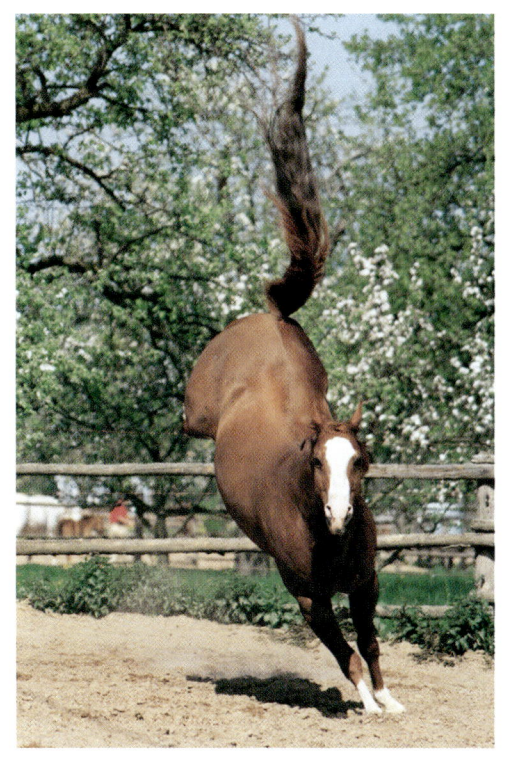

53. Injury is also possible in the paddock. By using PPS you can warm up your horse in the stable, as seen in Figs. 9 and 10.

5.1. THE WARM-UP IN CONNECTION WITH PPS

Responsible riders attach great importance to warming up the horse. The reason? To loosen the muscles slowly before making greater demands on them. Take a dressage rider for example; he strives for exceptional flowing movement; this is not possible when the horse is not sufficiently warmed up. The horse needs time for his movements to become smoother. A sensitive rider can feel this change and knows when to start with the real work.

What exactly happens when a horse slowly warms up? The muscles stretch and relax during the movement, positive stimulants enter the body, and the circulation of blood speeds up until the "machine runs at maximum". Unfortunately movement alone cannot relieve serious tension.

What if you use PPS? The pressure from your fingers triggers the release of stimulants and blood flow – exactly as if the horse has been warmed up in riding. With PPS you can detect strains and unease before riding, and deal with the problem immediately, supplementing the warm-up and preparing the horse for optimum performance.

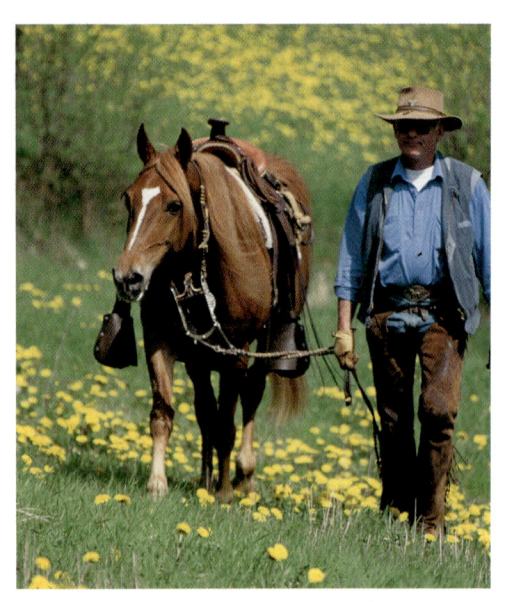

Additional information and gymnastic exercises

54. Unfortunately few riders and horses take time to cool off properly. Fifteen minutes should be the minimum time.

5.2. IMPORTANT AND OFTEN FORGOTTEN: COOLING DOWN

How much do you actually know about cooling down after a ride? A very important part of athletic training is the concluding round of walk.

It is surprising how little is known about this phase of training, which is possibly the most significant when it comes to injuries and strains. Unlike the warm up, it is difficult to decide when a horse has cooled off sufficiently. This can be influenced by various factors: is it warm or cold? What condition is your horse in? Has he been ill lately, etc?

The muscles become tired from exercise, waste products are deposited, so the horse has to move around slowly to get his body temperature down to normal, and the circulatory system must be given time to remove the waste products; this will lessen the tightness of the muscles.

When it is cold out, feel around the horse's ear, as in Figure 55. This gives a good indication of the horse's temperature.

It is not easy to ride around until a really wet horse has completely dried off; they prefer to be brushed and then moved again. Within a few minutes the hair will lie flat; simply groom the horse again.

Why not just throw a rug over the horse? There are rugs that can let the sweat evaporate, as long as you do not let the horse stand still but keep it moving.

55. This is an excellent way to test the body temperature of your horse, especially in winter.

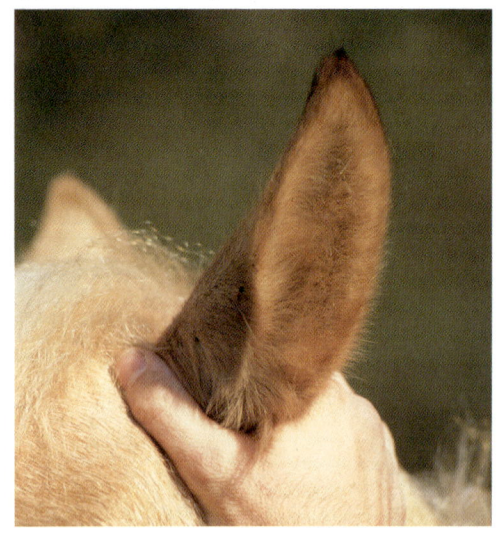

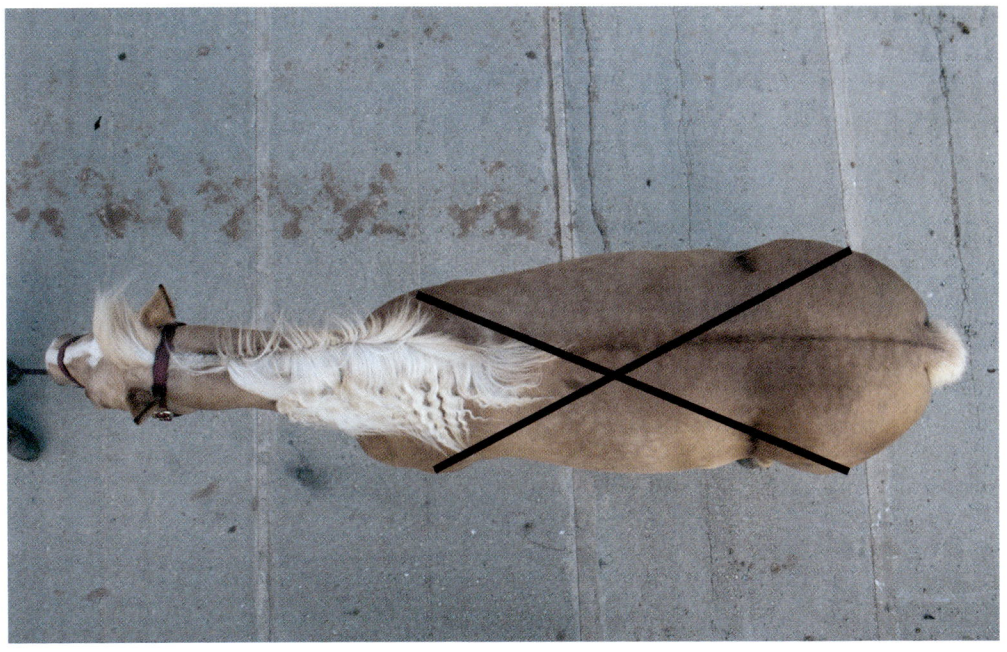

Additional information and gymnastic exercises

56. The horses's legs function diagonally with each other, left fore with right hind, and the other way round. When there is tension in the left fore, the right hind must work harder and is thus itself more prone to strain. This should be considered with targeted exercises.

5.3. EXERCISES TO BUILD THE MUSCLES

Gymnastic exercises that build muscle and help relieve tension are a further component of our "hot line to the horse". Regular exercises that build the muscles are needed to eliminate the tension and to ensure the effectiveness of PPS, as conveyed at the beginning of this book.

Once you have eliminated tension by using PPS, it is important that the relieved muscles work in harmony with the others. I would like to introduce an exercise to target the areas that have been under strain. First of all I would like to remind you of the relation between parts of the horse's body and the movement in it: the legs function diagonally with each other, the left fore with the right hind and the other way round. Where there is tension in the left fore, the right hind must work harder and is therefore more prone to strain.

Remember the spider's web, where all the muscles connect with each other and a single tense muscle draws all the other into despair as well.

Most of the problems have their origin in the muscles that have been tested

Additional information and gymnastic exercises

and which show the most severe reactions; they have been under strain the longest.

Now on to the exercise: you need continuous movement that makes a demand on the muscle that has, due to the tension, been underdeveloped and therefore grown weaker without putting the neighbouring muscles under strain. Working on a slope has proven the most successful for this. Naturally it means effort on your part as well!

To have any effect it should be performed at least three times a week, with the extra advantage that it also prepares the horse for the next season.

I will explain the exercise for a horse that shows specific reactions in the left hind or right fore. In order to train the right hind and the matching left fore, simply change the exercise by starting on the other side.

The reason will be quite clear; however it is preferable to train both sides at the same time. Lead the horse slowly from the bottom right to the top left of the slope (Figure 57).

Leading the horse slowly up the slope needs more strength on the part of the rider – you too will build a few muscles in the process…

The left hind must carry approximately three-quarters of the weight in this way. Naturally the horse will notice this extra load and try to straighten himself to go straight up the hill, thereby loading the hind legs equally. Use a crop initially to keep the horse moving diagonally up the slope (Figure 58). At the top of the slope, turn around and walk down the same way; this time it is the right fore that has to carry three-quarters of the weight. Within a few weeks you will notice that it is easier for the horse (and yourself!).

Normal training of the horse can follow this exercise. The horse will be exhausted at first, but regular PPS and this exercise will soon make a remarkable difference in your horse's well-being and performance.

The exercise in Figures 57 to 59 is based on a slope of 100m. Up and down will come to 200m, and count as one repetition. If your slope is shorter, do more repetitions. Once the dexterity on both sides becomes equal, you can do corresponding work on both sides, say five times each side.
If you notice one side to be weaker on going up or down, you can fall back on the proportion of 6:4 once more.

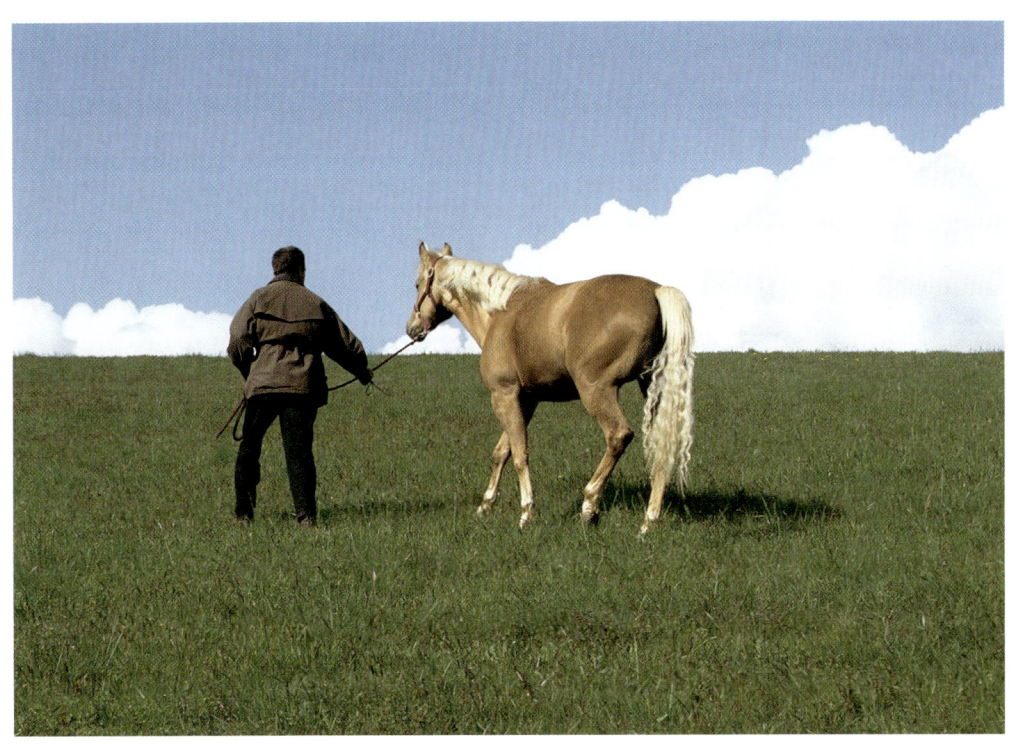

Additional information and gymnastic exercises

57. Lead the horse six times from bottom right to top left of the slope. This trains the left hind and right fore the most when this is the side with the most obvious problems. The other side must be balanced by leading the horse four times from bottom left to top right of the slope.

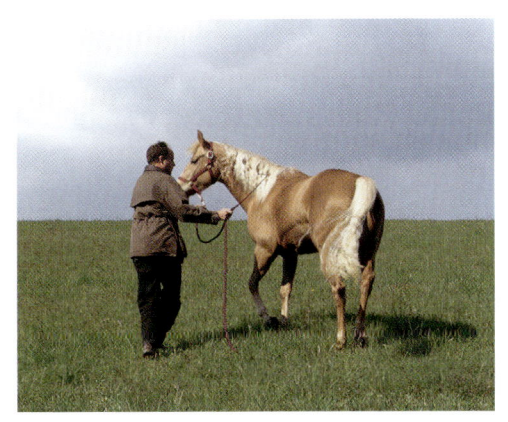

58. When the horse tries to make it easy by going straight up the slope, use a crop to keep it on the diagonal track.

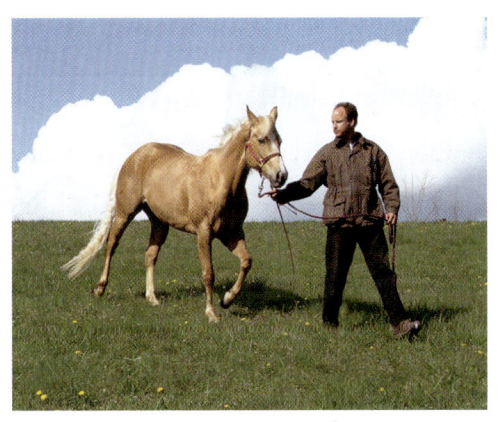

59. Walking down the slope. Within six to eight weeks you will notice that the muscles are more even on both sides. Continue for another two weeks with the 6:4 proportions as in Fig. 59, and then change to 5:5.

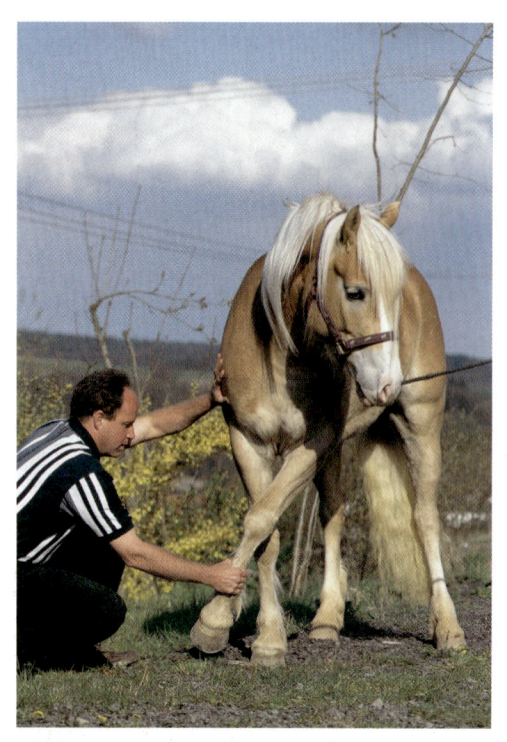

Additional information and gymnastic exercises

60. Crossing the forelimb. Cross one leg over the other. Carefully pull the knee to the front and hold this position for 10 seconds. As a complete exercise you can cross the hind leg as well.

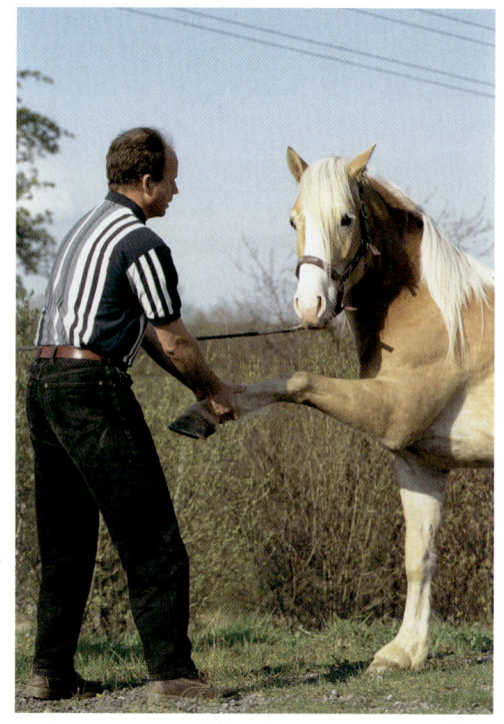

61. Raising the forelimb. Raise the forelimb to a 90-degree angle, then hold this position for 10 seconds. Take care to keep your own back straight.

5.4. STRETCHING: USEFUL GYMNASTIC EXERCISES FOR YOUR HORSE

Have you ever seen how a cat wakes up and stretches itself in all directions? In all my years of treating horses, and every

62. Hind leg stretch. Carefully pull the hind leg until it is fully stretched. With tension in regions 5, 6, or 7 it will not be possible to stretch the leg completely. Proceed slowly should the horse attempt to pull the leg away. Wait until the horse relaxes and try again. Be patient – this takes practice! Hold the end position for 5 seconds.

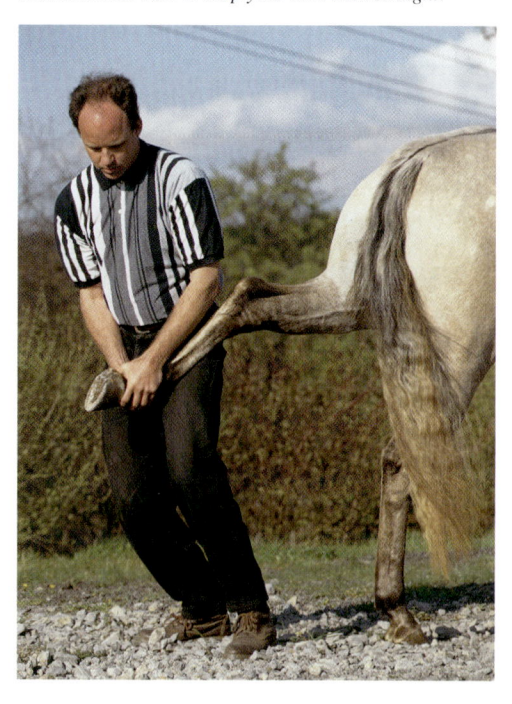

Additional information and gymnastic exercises

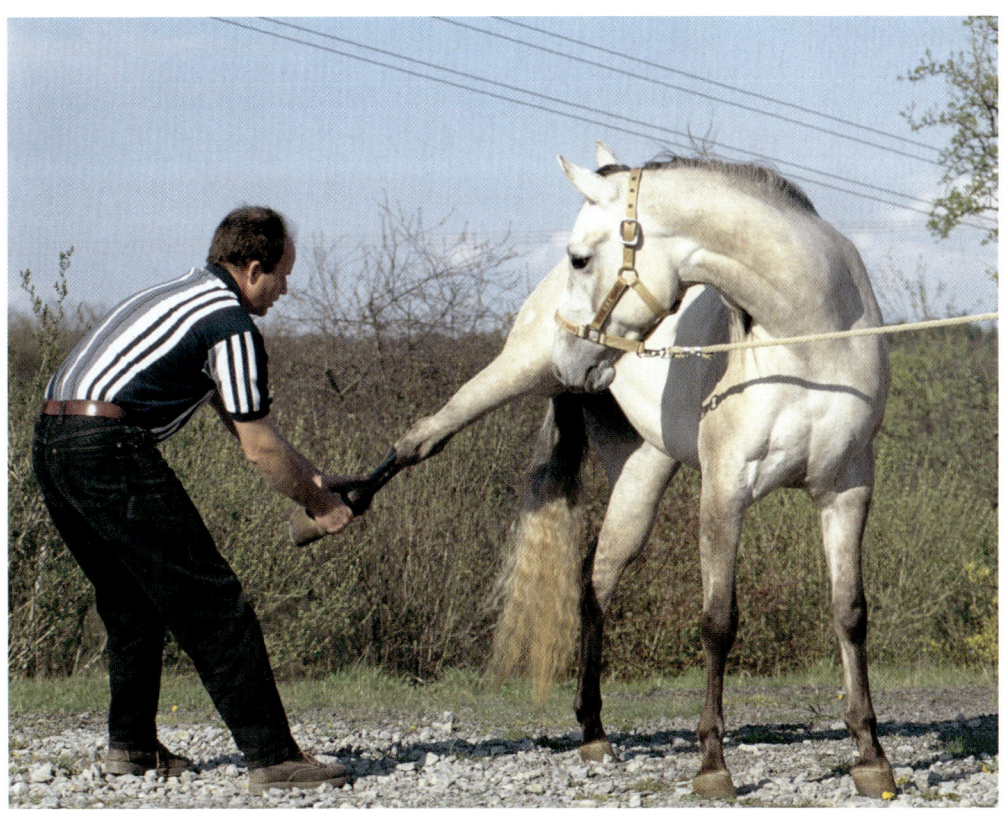

63. Hind leg to the side. Carefully pull the hind leg to the side as far as it can go. It may look peculiar, but you can raise the leg about as high as the hock. Hold this position for 5 seconds.

64/65. Hind leg to the front. Pull the hoof of the hind leg to the front (67). It is possible to stretch to three-quarters of the way to the front leg (65). Tension in region 8 makes this very difficult for the horse. Do not keep your head above the hoof and notice how I hold the hoof; this way I will be hurled out of harm's way if the horse kicks. Hold this position for 5 seconds.

64

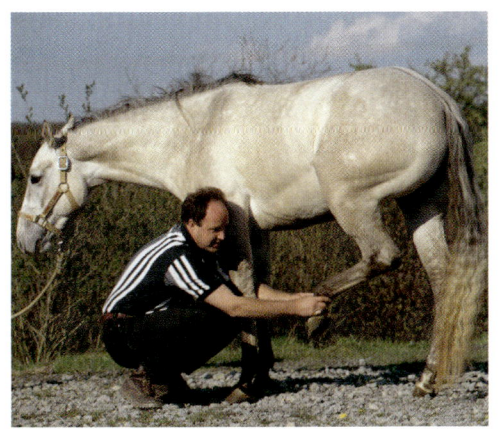

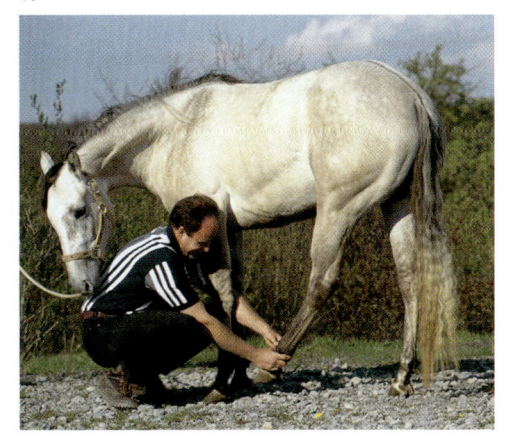

65

Additional information and gymnastic exercises

so often a dog, I have never been asked to treat a cat with tension. These animals have their own stretching programme that keeps them supple, and they seldom suffer from strains.

In a previous chapter, oedema was discussed; the fluid in the tissue thickens within four to five months and influences the range of movement in the muscle-tendon unit, encouraging tension that you notice when riding. It is possible to press oedema out of muscles by stretching them, similar to pressing toothpaste from a tube, as long as the oedema has not hardened. You can achieve a great deal with selective stretching when loosening hard regions with PPS. Start your stretching regime with the legs and move on to the back and neck. If the horse tries to avoid the stretch you must take it very slowly and do a little more every time until you reach the maximum stretch. Work gently and with patience to help the horse get used to these unusual movements!

Stretching should be done three times a day if possible. Remember, practice makes perfect!

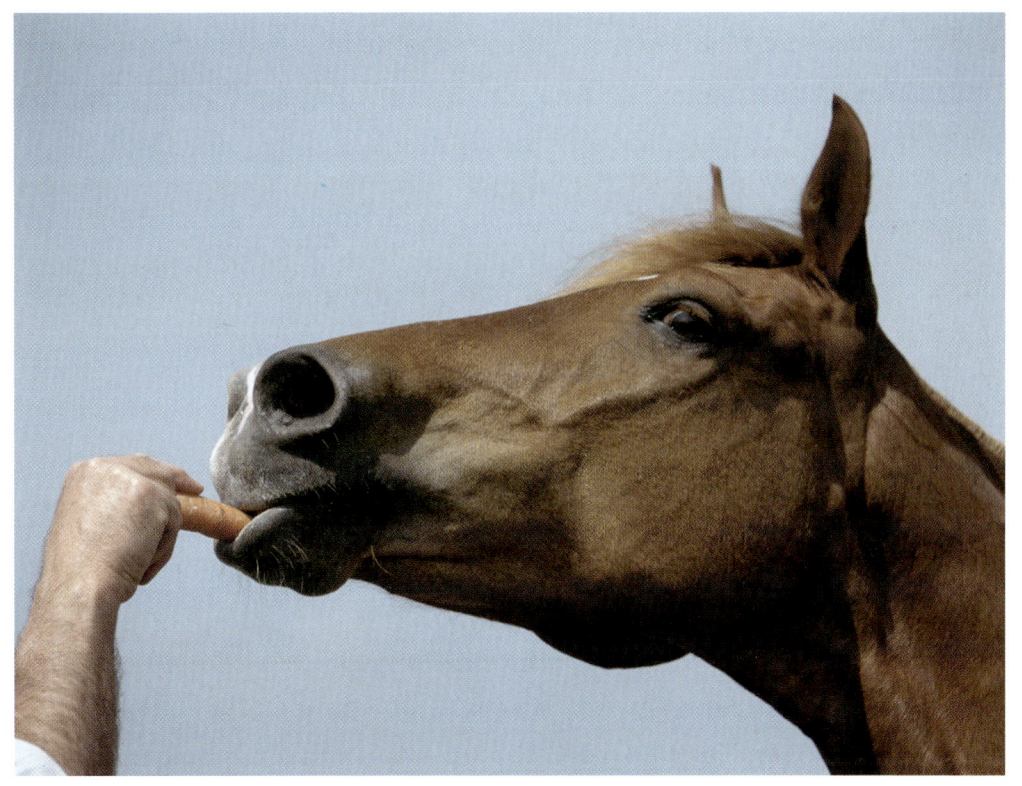

Additional information and gymnastic exercises

66. Horses love carrots (bananas as well, by the way…) Let us capitalise on this!

5.5
THE CARROT TRICK

Flexibility of the neck, shoulders and forelimbs is increased with the carrot trick. This exercise is fun for both the horse and trainer; the horse gets a reward for stretching and the trainer can see daily progress in the flexibility of the horse.

You only need a carrot!

You must have observed your horse scratching the back of his head with the hoof of his hind leg, or using his teeth to

> A highly important point in this exercise is to start and finish with the stretch in Figures 67/68. Take care that the horse's back is straight and the head bends on a straight line.
> The result of the carrot trick over a period of time is that the stretched neck and back will slot into place in a relaxed and accurate way.
> This exercise completes the PPS in a sensible way.

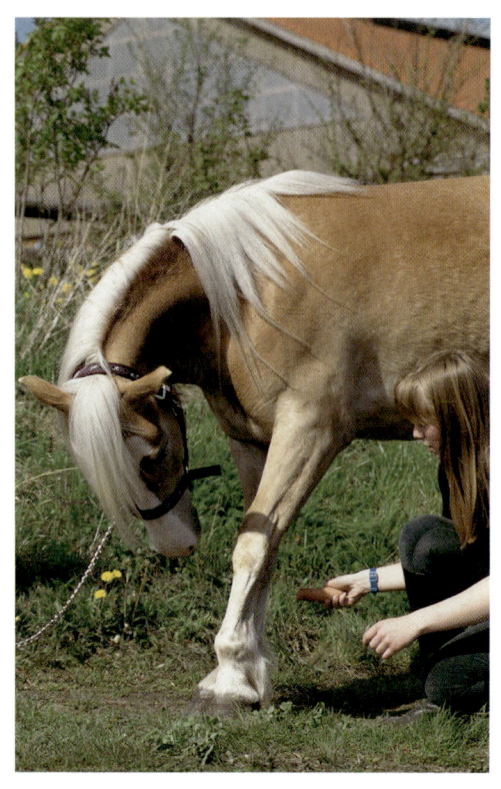

Additional information and gymnastic exercises

67. Carrot stretching. Lead the horse's head and neck through the forelegs with the carrot.

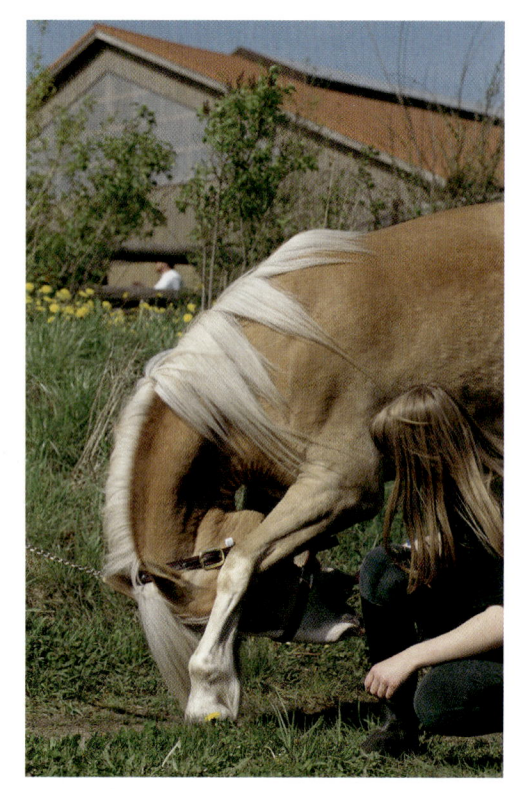

68. When the head is properly on the chest, let the horse bite the carrot. Take care that the back is straight in doing this!

get to an itchy spot on his hind leg or croup.

These exercises encourage corresponding agility and it is recommended to do these just before feeding. The carrot will lure the head and neck in the desired direction, thus stretching individual muscles and loosening the vertebrae at the same time.

Once the horse has learned the different positions, he will get hold of the carrot without a problem. Within a few attempts you will find it easier to use a long thin carrot rather than a short fat one; after all, you would like to have your fingers at the end of it…

Although some of these carrot exercises look peculiar, with a bit of practice every horse can comprehend them. The exercise is to stretch the vertebrae of the neck (Figure 67) and also stretch the vertebrae to both sides (Figures 69/70/71). Take your time when doing this exercise!

Take three weeks to reach the final position if necessary, slowly increasing

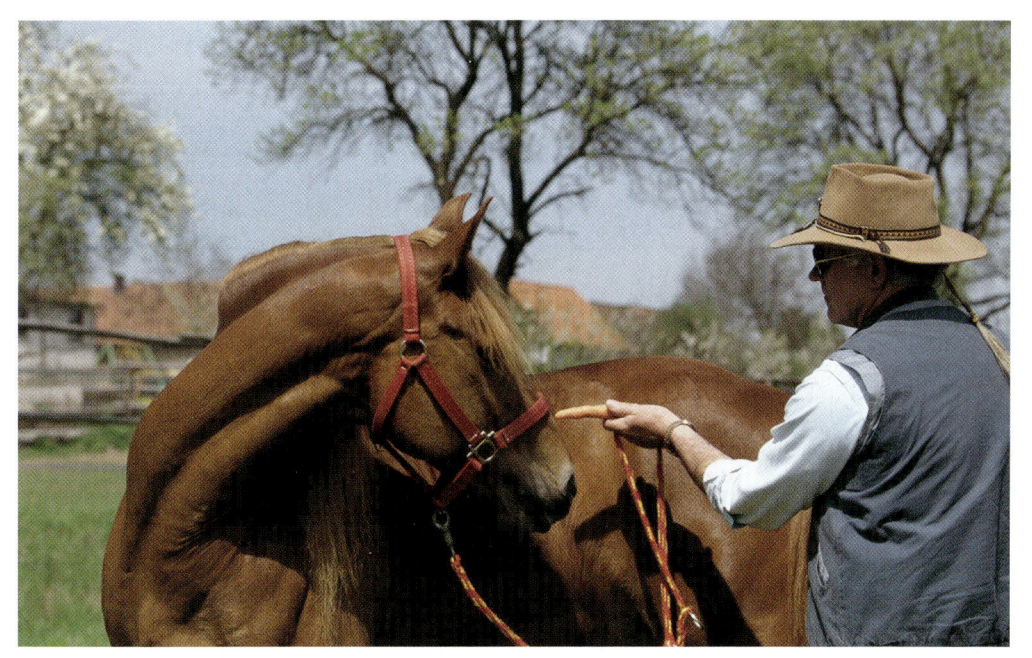

Additional information and gymnastic exercises

69. Carrot stretch – first week. Lead the horse to this position for a week and let the horse bite a piece of the carrot. This is not easy for the horse, you only want him to bend his neck and stretch the relevant muscles. Remember to do this on both sides and end with the stretch in Figures 67/68.

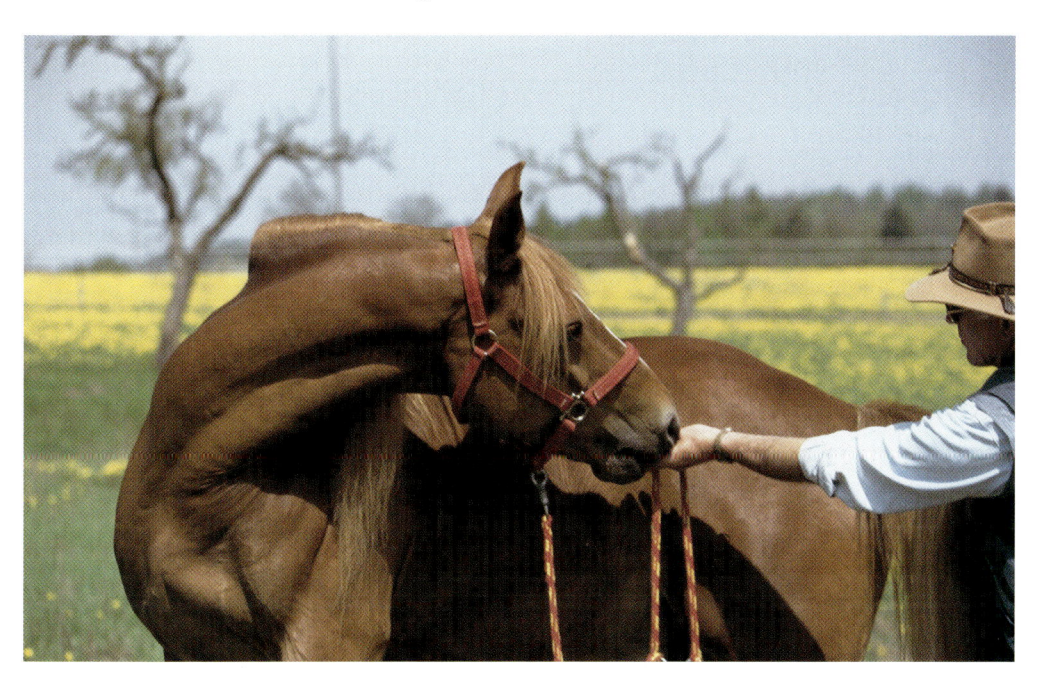

70. Carrot stretch – second week. In the second week the muscles will be able to stretch further. The exercise might seem easy, but the muscles do need time to reach maximum extension. See that your horse stretches only his neck, and not his body. Remember the exercise of Figures 67/68.

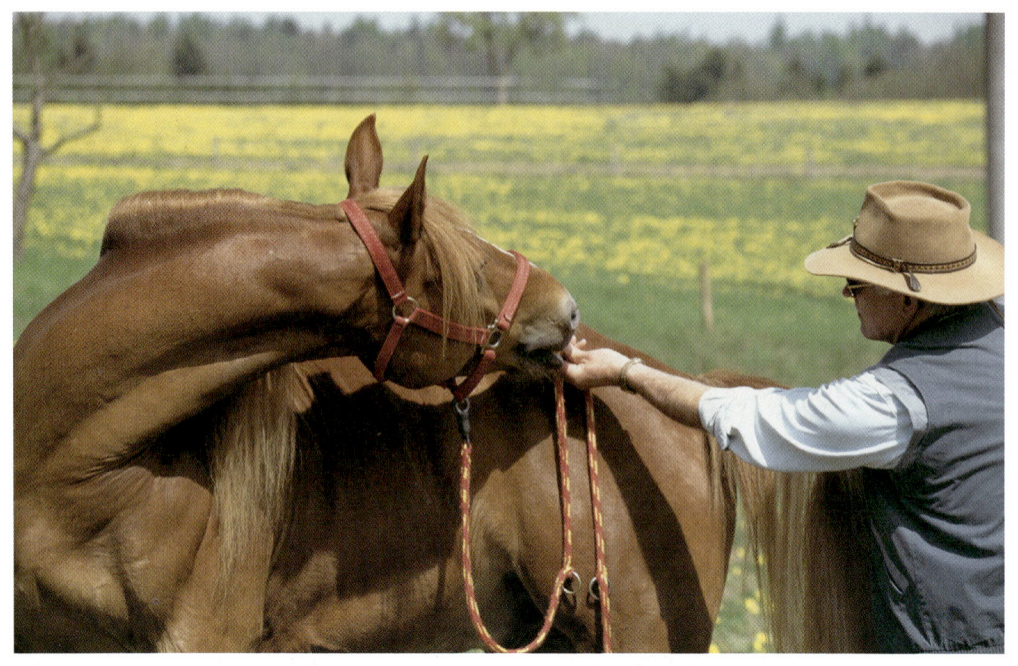

Additional information and gymnastic exercises

71. Carrot stretch – third week. In the third week you can request the maximum stretch. You have given the horse enough time to get accustomed to this unusual action.

the demand, and only proceed as far as shown in the photographs!

I hope you really give your horse three weeks to stretch to the maximum; after all, you probably would not be able to do the splits in so short a time! After three weeks you will soon notice the difference in elasticity in the horse's neck, shoulders and forelegs.

This exercise, together with PPS, can rid your horse of tension and improve his well-being.

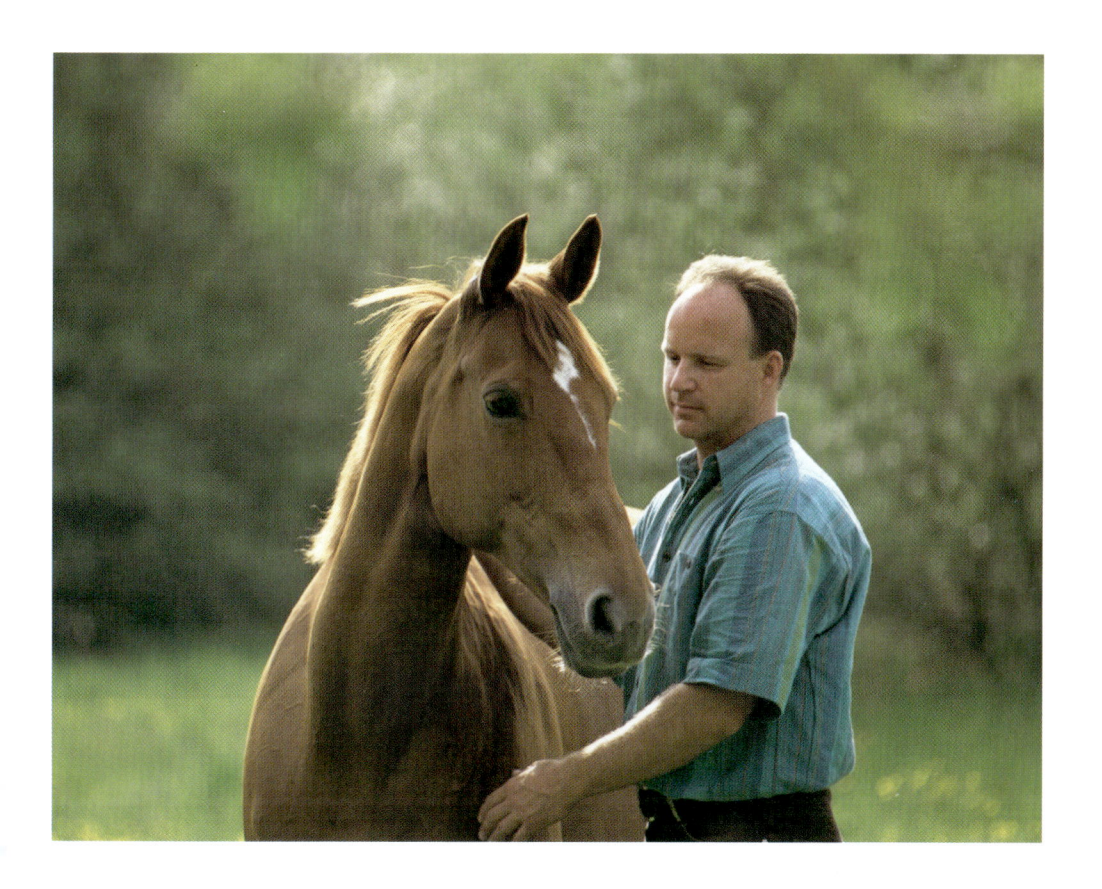

CONCLUSION

I know that you derive a lot of pleasure from your horse and you are aware of your great responsibility, or you would not have bought this book. Many of you are experienced horse people; others may perhaps only ride occasionally, or own a horse for only a short time.

Horses only seem undemanding because they adapt to us. However, they do need fair and consistent treatment in order to unfold their power and personality to us. Real relaxation can only come from inside the horse, but let us be realistic: you cannot expect your horse to be relaxed when you are not capable of doing it yourself! Neither you nor your horse will function well when compelled to do something.

Conclusion

There are people all over the world that get along faultlessly with their horses, and all have their own little tricks for doing so. The "hot line to the horse", the work with PPS, is my own personal way of working with horses, which I have attempted to share with you in this book. I hope by doing so that I have stimulated your interest in PPS, thereby enabling you to ride your horse with more satisfaction in a more relaxed way in the future.

A big thank you goes to everyone who has supported and motivated me in the writing of this book. This includes those involved in taking the photographs, and the Old Mountain Ranch.

A special thank you to the tireless efforts of Helmut and Adelheid Lauber, as well as Christiane Slawik. Without them this book would probably not exist.

To conclude I would like to thank the members of my family who staunchly influenced me with regard to horses:

Bessy Olson
Lenus Olson
Donald Olson
Shawn Olson
Matt Miller